Praise for Jerry L

MW01093075

"Over the years, I have had the opportunity to stay informed by Jerry Lynch, information that makes a difference in helping me and my athletes reach our potential. Our minds and hearts are in harmony. You will learn the why and how from Jerry's latest book, COACHING WITH HEART."

Phil Jackson, former coach of Chicago Bulls and L.A.Lakers
Eleven-time NBA World Champion

"Jerry is a wise and trusted friend who happens to be one of the nation's top authorities on leadership and coaching in sports. His input has had a very positive influence in helping me and other coaches at Carolina to create environments that inspire athletes to go the distance and reach their potential. This book will definitely make a difference in your coaching as well."

Anson Dorrance, head women's soccer coach, University North Carolina
Five-time National Coach of theYear
21 NCAA National Championships
Winningest women's soccer coach of all time

"Having played for several incredibly dynamic coaches during my career, I embrace Jerry Lynch's message in COACHING WITH HEART, a book about inspiration not just in sports but in life, family, goals, and desires. My favorite coaches were the ones who understood Jerry's ideals and strived to connect with me on a human level. That's what this book is all about."

Steve Kerr, former five-time NBA World Champion with Bulls and Spurs
Former GM for Phoenix Suns
NBA TV color commentator and analyst

"No other person has had more influence on my 36 years of coaching than Jerry Lynch. Whenever I need wisdom, insight, or inspiration I look to Dr. Lynch. His work never fails to address the truly essential elements of coaching, which is interacting from the heart. This book will light the match for you to keep strong relationships at the very core of your coaching."

Missy Foote, head women's lacrosse coach, women's AD at Middlebury College
6 NCAA National Championships
Seven-time National Coach of the Year
2012 USA Lacrosse Hall of Fame

"My success in Lacrosse and in life has been directly and positively influenced by the books, wisdom, and work of Dr. Jerry Lynch. His new book, COACHING WITH HEART, presents powerful strategies to help open all of our hearts as well as those of your athletes. This is a must read... the REAL deal."

Cindy Timchal, head lacrosse coach, US Naval Academy
8 NCAA National Lacrosse Championships
The winningest coach in Div.1 Lacrosse
National Lacrosse Hall of Fame

"Jerry Lynch is among the most influential sports psychologists of our time and his books should be on the shelf of every coach and leader. In his latest book, he offers insights that are inspirational and enduring, as well as stimulating and practical. Such an important contribution to the profession of coaching."

Dr. Cory Dobbs, President and CEO, The Academy of Sport Leadership.

"Jerry has had a profound positive influence in my personal and professional life for over 20 years. I have witnessed his work with numerous coaches and athletes achieve striking results. His leadership training, development of team culture, and coaching expertise is unparalleled and makes athletic and coaching experience even more compelling, relevant, and enjoyable."

Bob Hansen, head tennis coach at Middlebury College
34 NCAA team and individual National Championships, six-time National Coach of the Year and National Coach of the Decade 2000-2012

"At the University of North Carolina, we aim to exhaust the potential of our student athletes in the physical, emotional, and spiritual arenas of their lives. Jerry has been instrumental in helping us build an approach where we can coach and compete with heart while inspiring authentic growth in those we lead. COACHING WITH HEART will provide you with insight and wisdom from his years of experience, affording you the opportunity to kick your coaching up a few notches."

Jenny Levy, head women's lacrosse coach, University, North Carolina
4th Winningest active coach in Lacrosse
Six-time Final Four appearances
2013 National Champions

"Working with Dr. Lynch has helped my coaching and our culture to climb several notches in just two years. Our athletes, because of this growth in leadership, are competing at a whole new level. Coaching has become so much more enjoyable. We feel we are truly teaching our athletes to become leaders for life through sport. His 'way' is worth living every single day."

Kit Vela, head women's soccer coach, University New Mexico
Two-time Mountain West, Conference Champions

COACHING
WITH
HEART

Taoist Wisdom to Inspire, Empower, and Lead

Jerry Lynch, Ph.D.

Calligraphy By
Chungliang Al Huang

TUTTLE Publishing

Tokyo | Rutland, Vermont | Singapore

The Tuttle Story: "Books to Span the East and West"

Many people are surprised to learn that the world's largest publisher of books on Asia had its humble beginnings in the tiny American state of Vermont. The company's founder, Charles E. Tuttle, belonged to a New England family steeped in publishing.

Immediately after WW II, Tuttle served in Tokyo under General Douglas MacArthur and was tasked with reviving the Japanese publishing industry. He later founded the Charles E. Tuttle Publishing Company, which thrives today as one of the world's leading independent publishers.

Though a westerner, Tuttle was hugely instrumental in bringing a knowledge of Japan and Asia to a world hungry for information about the East. By the time of his death in 1993, Tuttle had published over 6,000 books on Asian culture, history and art—a legacy honored by the Japanese emperor with the "Order of the Sacred Treasure," the highest tribute Japan can bestow upon a non-Japanese.

With a backlist of 1,500 titles, Tuttle Publishing is more active today than at any time in its past—inspired by Charles Tuttle's core mission to publish fine books to span the East and West and provide a greater understanding of each.

Published by Tuttle Publishing, an imprint of Periplus Editions (HK) Ltd.

www.tuttlepublishing.com

Copyright © 2013 Jerry Lynch

Library of Congress Cataloging-in-Publication Data in process

ISBN 978-0-8048-4348-5

First edition
15 14 13   5 4 3 2 1   1309CP

Printed in Singapore

Distributed by

North America, Latin America & Europe
Tuttle Publishing
364 Innovation Drive
North Clarendon,
VT 05759-9436 U.S.A.
Tel: 1 (802) 773-8930
Fax: 1 (802) 773-6993
info@tuttlepublishing.com
www.tuttlepublishing.com

Asia Pacific
Berkeley Books Pte. Ltd.
61 Tai Seng Avenue #02-12
Singapore 534167
Tel: (65) 6280-1330
Fax: (65) 6280-6290
inquiries@periplus.com.sg
www.periplus.com

TUTTLE PUBLISHING® is a registered trademark of Tuttle Publishing, a division of Periplus Editions (HK) Ltd.

CONTENTS

Meeting Dean At The Dome

He has been called a "coaching legend" by the Basketball Hall of Fame. To athletes like Michael Jordan, James Worthy, Phil Ford, Sam Perkins, and others under his tutelage over a 37 year span, he is simply called "Coach." His name is Dean Smith, retired coach of men's basketball at the University of North Carolina.

I have been enamored with this icon, leader, mentor, and teacher-coach since his arrival in "Tar Heel Country" back in 1961. I loved basketball and I loved him: his coaching style, his athlete-centered approach, and his "way of being" on and off the court. He was, to me, what extraordinary coaching was all about. He was the quintessential leader of men. However, all of my perceptions about him were formed from afar, reading accounts about him in *Sports Illustrated*, observing him during games, and listening to others as they spoke fondly about this amazing legend. Yet, this was not enough for me. I desired to have an opportunity to know firsthand, in person, face to face, what this man was really like and to feel his presence, up close and personal, and perhaps get to really understand the essence of such a great man.

That opportunity fortuitously came to me exactly a year ago while I was working at the University of North Carolina with Jenny Levy, head coach of the women's lacrosse program. Basically, I followed Nike's advice and I "just did it." I meandered over to the Dean Smith Center, the basketball arena on campus affectionately called the "Dean Dome" and showed up to see if I could reserve an appointment for some future date out of respect for his stature and busy schedule. To my surprise and delight, his secretary of several decades (this should tell you a lot about him) said to me: "If you can wait just a minute Dr. Lynch, I will tell him you are here. I am sure he'd love to meet you." She returned within a minute, closely followed by my coaching hero.

I was a bit shocked and awestruck by his presence. I wasn't "prepared" for this. What do I say? What will he say? How will I be? A bit nervous and apprehensive, a normal response to such a surprise, we sat down together and all my questions, concerns, and worries dissipated as we began to talk. He was gentle, kind, respectful, caring, interested, loving, trusting, warm, encouraging, genuine, humble, modest, and filled with integrity, all of the essential spiritual qualities of one who coaches with heart. As I left his office following our unexpected 45 minute conversation I was overwhelmed with love and emotion. It was at that precise moment that I understood what extraordinary coaching was all about and why so many have admired this amazing human being. Had he asked me to lick the dust off the basketball court so that the team could practice, I would have done it instantly. With his heart-directed approach I would be sure to go the distance. I was so inspired and empowered during this session by his warmth, caring, and respect that I felt compelled and motivated to write my next book, *Coaching with Heart: Tao Wisdom to Inspire, Empower, and Lead.*

OPEN MIND, RECEPTIVE HEART

As we begin the journey of coaching with heart together, I want to encourage you to maintain an open mind and heart to new possibilities, directions, and ways to be in this extraordinary profession of coaching. I present in this book a host of suggestions for contemplation, not indoctrination. The *Tao Te Ching* makes this poignant observation:

> *To be empty we can be full yet*
> *To be full we stay empty.*
> *Abundance is within Emptiness.*

Most of us in the profession of coaching believe that we, as teachers, must know all. Wise coaches know they don't know all which makes it easy to begin to learn. Taoist leaders and sages claim that one who does not know actually knows, and one who knows really does not know. Consider the classic Zen story about a pompous professor who goes to the master to learn about Zen Buddhism. The Zen master invites him for tea, and to enlighten him he pours the tea until the cup is overflowing. The professor protests and the master gently explains to him, "Exactly. Your knowledge is already spilling over so how can I offer you anymore?"

It feels good to be an "empty cup." As a heart-directed coach, consider the practice of remaining open and empty to position yourself to receive new ways of being. The *Tao* warrior coach actually strives to "appear" less knowledgeable than he or she is, and, in the process, commits fewer errors and mistakes having less pressure to live up to someone he or she is not.

This is the essence of emptiness, pregnant with potential and containing many more possibilities. It is an exciting place where anything can happen and usually does. It is a sacred space where the "tea of learning" can be poured into an area of emptiness that contains all potential.

The Chinese symbols for emptiness depict an empty vessel to be filled and refilled as long as the "fertile mind" is maintained. If you remain open and receptive to what this book brings to you there is the chance that your coaching career will be dynamically long, exciting, fruitful, fun-filled, and deeply satisfying. Be an open vessel, fill up, and enjoy the journey you are about to begin.

CALLIGRAPHIC ART

Speaking of Chinese symbols, notice how they are interspersed throughout this book? The cover calligraphy itself is a symbol meaning "having love in your heart," a concept that immediately sets the tone for all that will follow. I want to deeply acknowledge my dear friend and co-author of several of my books, Chungliang Al Huang, for his continued support and love as demonstrated with his beautiful calligraphy. I am honored and privileged to have him contribute to my work once again. His Chinese symbols visually show the kinetic power of the dancing spirit and have become a unique brand for our books as well as my nationwide and international business, Way of Champions. The aesthetic beauty of his artistic contribution reinforces the theme, quality, and impact of this book upon all of us. I am forever grateful for his guidance in helping me to better grasp the essence of the Tao. Peruse more of his work at livingtao.org.

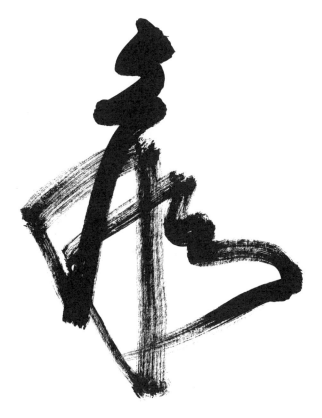

INTRODUCTION

Sea Change With A Dancing Heart

For the past 34 years, I have been fortunate, honored, and privileged to be invited into the inner sanctums of collegiate and professional athletic programs to coach the coaches and athletes to believe that they can be something other than ordinary. I have written and published eleven books, all from this experience, reflecting what I have learned from thousands of these great spirits who have opened their hearts, allowing me to focus on making a difference in their lives. Gathering stories, collecting observations, gaining insight, and expanding wisdom, I am here to say that I notice a huge paradigm shift taking place in the profession of coaching; athletes are demanding positive relationship change with their leaders. Such an historic "sea change" tells me that those being coached are seeking a change of heart from those doing the coaching to a more dynamic, multifaceted approach. Still interested in the necessity of developing and learning the essential skills, tactics, and strategies of their sport, the athletes also seem to desire being taught this knowledge in environments that are marinated in respect, trust, love, compassion, and integrity. In other words, while they care about what you know as their coach (Xs and Os), they also want to know that you care (inspire and empower). In a sense, they are asking their leaders to "dance" between both axes of coaching, to coach with heart, thus the genesis of the title of this book.

THE DANCING HEART PROCESS

In this new book, I offer practical, useable, and dynamic concepts for positive change and success in the ever-shifting landscape of the profession of coaching. Coaches who are successful in sport are beginning to realize that they need to win the "relationship game" and the athletic game will take care of itself. What they are discovering is that coaching is ultimately a "path of heart," a relationship dance between athlete and coach, and the counterpart dance between teaching the athletes skill-sets for optimal performance coupled with the wisdom of inspiration that will empower the athletes to "go the distance" in sports and life.

First, we have the relationship dance, which in Chinese is called Wu Tao. Here is the dance between giving and receiving, receiving and giving. To be a good coach, mentor, and teacher you must be a good student and learn what needs to be known from the student (the athlete) in order to teach them what they must learn. In this dancing relationship, each individual is interdependent—forming a bond of equal fulfillment, love, and respect in a harmonious atmosphere of openness, communication, and loyalty. Each person involved in this mutually beneficial dance, genuinely experiences the gifts each has to offer. This fluid, rhythmic, flowing, and dancing union between coach and athlete, serving and sharing together for the greater good of all, is an extraordinary process to behold. It is the cornerstone of the "coaching with heart" process. True learning and development take place in all arenas of life when giving and receiving are intrinsic to each member of the relationship.

Second, extraordinary leadership and coaching involves a dance between two distinct axes. The first axis demands the devotion of the leader's time and energy to performance management, strategic planning, and a myriad of other "Xs and Os" preparatory exercises. While these aspects of leadership are absolutely essential to the coaching piece, there is yet another axis that is a willing partner in this second dance. This other axis in this union is spiritually based—one that is related to the first dance, Wu Tao, and by definition enables you to inspire and empower those being led. Herein lies the essence of this book.

The challenge at this point is for all of us to discover ways to dance together, to create safe environments and develop relationships of the heart. This book serves as a template to help us learn to dance with heart with those we lead by cultivating environments where hearts *can* dance; where teaching and learning is a dance between giving and receiving; where we, as leaders, can perfect the essential absolutes of love, inspiration, compassion, respect, understanding, and integrity while helping concurrently to develop the skill sets so necessary to perform the tasks at hand. When we influence and dance with others in this way, they feel valued and perform more optimally in an encouraging environment, free of fear and intimidation. With an increase of love, compassion, and spirituality, people become happy, trust and respect deepen, and the results and outcomes are greatly enhanced. Simply stated, when we coach with a dancing heart and develop relationships like this, those we lead are more joyful, cooperative, and happy and therefore work harder; when anyone works harder, results and outcomes usually improve.

Additionally, athletes in such environments will begin to prepare, practice, play, compete, and live with heart themselves. Your coaching becomes the model used by all those under your guidance for their own personal leadership on and off the field.

I am aware also that this book could have a significant impact on the direction of coaching educators in a time when athletics is experiencing an influx of leaders, a new generation who desire to master both the Xs and Os of their game and the inspiration and empowerment pieces as well. This book will change the focus of coaching, your understanding of athletes and those you lead.

Another valuable function of this book is how it can facilitate your progress of getting to know yourself better, to cultivate your inner guidance system called intuition, to influence others by example and attitude, and to lead and

coach by guiding rather than forcing others to comply, building resentment and rebellion; better to create environments
of loyalty, trust, respect, and cooperation where resistance
and counterforce are virtually eliminated, while instilling a
strong sense of personal power in those you lead. You will
discover that by being such a heart-directed leader, you will
empower others and, simultaneously, gain power yourself.
Like electricity, the more energy and love you conduct, the
more you receive. In truth, you never need to display power.
Others just feel it and respect it because such an extraordinary leader radiates and emanates personal power.

The principles, strategies, wisdom, and overall lessons of
this book will guide you to develop a more athlete-centered
approach for those under your guidance, thus helping you
to master the art of highly effective, enlightened, and extraordinary leadership.

This book is written for the entire population of people
and professionals who desire to become inspirational and
empowering coaches, helping those they lead to grow and
develop into their full human potential and capacity. Such
coaches in athletics, business, education, church congrega-
tions, military organizations, and parents of athletic-orient-
ed kids are but a few of those targeted populations that could
benefit from this book. The wisdom and lessons within these
pages offer to all of us concepts, strategies, and tools for inspiring and empowering relationships in all walks of life. It
is a book designed to help you be in position to accelerate
the process of readiness for those whom we lead, who hesitate to move forward even though they desire to do so.

Think of this book as a commitment to change, transform, improve, and optimize the effective skill-set you al-

ready possess. We all feel from time to time that something is missing from our repertoire and we need to "rock the boat." Sometimes we feel stagnant or on a plateau and wish to take our performance to a higher level. Perhaps we want to get a stronger sense of purpose or motivation and have a different success experience, one that does not rely on outcomes and results. This just may be the book to nudge you along the path, requiring all of us to think outside-the-box, in order to coach with a dancing heart.

AVENUES OF WISDOM

There are two ways, essentially, for each of us to accrue wisdom in our lives. The first is painless: learning from the teachings of others. The second is painful: learning from the experience of our journeys in life. To accomplish the task of writing this book, I will intersperse both avenues of wisdom, alternating between wisdom from my professional calling and the wisdom of sacred books written over 25 centuries ago for leaders, generals, and heads of state in ancient China. The three major parts of this book will combine Wisdom to Inspire, Wisdom to Empower, and Wisdom of the Watercourse Way, the *Tao* itself.

SACRED CALLING

I have been working in the coaching professions for 34 years. During this period of time, I have established a consultancy that is unique, stimulating, practical, and game-changing, aimed at instilling the principles of leadership learned from extraordinary coaches and athletes.

When I give it some thought, I really haven't had a job during any of these years. Instead I have had a "sacred calling," honorable and privileged work of serving and giving to others where my focus has been on making a difference rather than making a living. The funny thing about that is the "making a difference" approach has provided me with making an extraordinary living. There's an important lesson here for all of us who attempt to reverse the process.

It has been a joyful, sacred calling thus far, one of learning, growing, and expanding, and filled with much passion and love, a path of endless self-discovery, revelations, openings, and epiphanies along the way. It has enabled me to experience 29 National Championship teams and write this, my eleventh book on the subject. I agree with the observation of Cervantes when he said: "The journey is better than the inn." And, I am not even halfway there. I have so, so much more to learn and many miles to go before I rest.

SACRED BOOKS

In Chinese, the word that best defines and epitomizes extraordinary leadership and coaching with a dancing heart is Jingshen, a Mandarin concept meaning to instill spirit, vitality, chi, passion, and personal power in those you lead.

To achieve Jingshen, the art of implementing ways to inspire and empower others, not only do I use my wisdom from my calling but I adapt the timeless lessons on leadership from several ancient sacred Chinese books, one of which is the Tao Te Ching, the most widely published book in the world aside from the Bible and a source of spiritual strength for centuries. It was written 26 hundred years ago, ostensibly by Lao-Tzu, a Taoist sage, for all who were in positions of leadership at that time and who possessed the potential to influence, inspire, and empower others in a strong, positive, and productive way. Each of the 81 verses contained within this classic offer ageless leadership lessons, principles, suggestions, and strategies for effective guidance that speak directly to one of our most challenging professions, athletic coaching. These lessons help to cultivate ideal relationships between you and your athletes while guiding them to go the distance in athletics and life.

In addition to this, these practical verses of sagely advice give insight into a more "natural way"; the way coaching and leadership were meant to be, in harmony with nature. For example, the *Tao Te Ching* talks about the power (TE) of a leader or coach to serve others from a place of love, caring, and spirituality, rather than the power over others by resorting to force and manipulation. This is the power you have to influence and encourage athletes to discover their motivation within, to have courage, commitment, integrity, perseverance, patience, selflessness, and be fearless. When this happens, there is a heightened sense of purpose, meaning, and relevance to what they do which happens to be the essence of motivation. The Chinese calligraphic symbol for *Tao* is made up of a head, signifying wisdom, and a foot, representing walking—literally translated it means "walking the way of wisdom."

If you are anything like me, you want to kick it up a few notches in your coaching. The wisdom of the *Tao Te Ching* will help you to do just that as you experience significant change, improvement, and growth in addition to what you already have mastered from years of good work. The leadership lessons from the *Tao Te Ching* are a compelling way to get the most out of what you do. This wisdom, along with the wisdom from other Chinese sources, will help you to begin to understand the essence of extraordinary coaching, guiding, mentoring, and teaching not only for your work but for the bigger picture of life in all arenas of performance.

I'm excited and eager to dive in and begin the journey. This book is written in the spirit of giving to each of you, all that I have learned from so many others wiser than myself. I am like a hole in a flute where the breath of these great spirits comes through to you.

The following are several specific examples of what *Coaching with Heart* will help you to create and cultivate in your heart-directed culture:

- spark the flames of enthusiasm, excitement, and inspiration that flicker in all athletes
- encourage athletes to win the inner battles for success in all of life
- create environments that are emotionally safe, without blame and judgment
- enable athletes to realize their full, expansive capacity in sports and life
- nurture team cohesion, harmony, and unity of purpose, one heart, one soul, one goal
- gain the dedication, trust, loyalty, love, and appreciation of all those whom you lead
- communicate so that athletes will listen to you and you to them
- permit risk and help others learn the lessons of failure for sport and life

- model powerful humanistic styles of leadership
- resolve conflict more peacefully and effectively
- create more joy, happiness, and fulfillment for athletes, helping them to perform at higher levels
- cultivate independence, interdependence, and confidence in those you lead
- encourage athletes to turn to you in times of crisis, rather than to outsiders or drugs
- nurture self-esteem in others and in yourself
- be respectful and sensitive to athletes' needs
- express anger or irritations without causing emotional damage
- become more accepting, flexible, and balanced in your coaching and in your life in general
- create a culture of winning and excellence in sports and life in general
- teach those you lead to prepare, plan, play, and compete with the heart of a warrior
- win the relationship game before winning the athletic game
- step outside the box and be more creative and dynamic in your coaching
- develop ways to inspire and empower others to find inner motivation to go the distance.

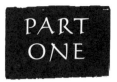

PART
ONE

WISDOM TO INSPIRE

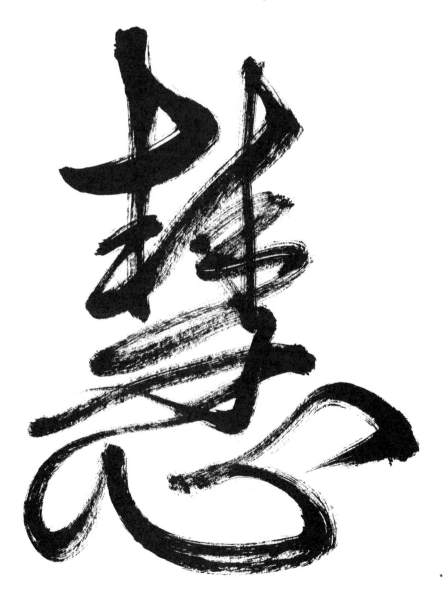

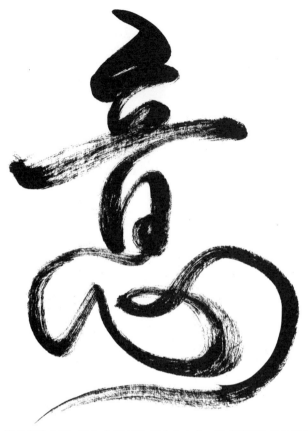

LEARNING EMOTIONAL INTELLIGENCE

The late great national championship coach Jim Valvano once said that "most people work by going to an office, I've been blessed…I get to coach." Having coached in some capacity for the past 34 years, I also feel blessed. If you are a coach, manager, mentor, parent, or leader in any arena of life—or aspire to become one—you are very fortunate and blessed as well. Coaching, I believe, is not a job; it is a most important calling, a sacred and vital activity where we have been given the fortunate opportunity and privilege to guide and mentor others in a nurturing, selfless, passionate environment, instilling in them the profound sense that they can be something other than ordinary. This calling may very well be one of the most compelling, significant, and honorable paths one could travel in a lifetime, the opportunity to cultivate and develop in others deep spiritual qualities of inspiration, excitement, fortitude, enthusiasm, loyalty, balance, courage, and self-reliance. Wow…can you imagine this? With such characteristics, those we coach experience authentic growth and development on the physical, emotional, and spiritual plane. This is not only possible but inevitable for anyone under the leadership of one who coaches with heart. In order to coach with heart we must nurture and develop in ourselves the same traits that we wish to instill in those we coach and lead. Traditionally, the work of a coach has been steeped in the left hemisphere of the brain, giving little or no attention to these heart-based attributes of their work and performance. I notice that good coaches are looking for ways to get help to coach with heart. They understand that without heart, a tone is set with a team, an organization, a family or individual that is often unloving, uncaring, and spiritless in a "results-driven" culture. Compare this to the cultures under the guidance of highly successful leaders and coaches such as a Dean Smith or a John Wooden and you will see that these brilliant leaders have much love in their coaching, not of the romantic nature but love demonstrated by deep caring, warmth, positive regard, respect, and compassion, all essential absolutes for coaching and leading with heart.

The good news is that these essential absolutes, this skill-set of interpersonal tools, is not innate and can be taught and learned with practice. According to the science of neuroplasticity, this skill-set is trainable; you can intentionally change how your brain functions to more positive, caring, and cooperative ways. This is what we will attempt to accomplish together in this book. These learned skills are often referred to as Emotional Intelligence (EI). All extraordinary coaches possess EI. In his bestselling book, *Search Inside Yourself*, Chade-Meng Tan talks extensively about EI as the essential ingredient that makes good leaders into great leaders. He points out that 80% of effective leadership qualities are made up from emotional intelligence and continues to emphasize that the most single, significant factor that differentiates top level leaders from the bottom is their handle on the interpersonal skill piece. It was what I experienced with Coach Dean Smith during my visit. EI makes all of us better, more effective leaders enabling each of us to make a difference with so many in our lives.

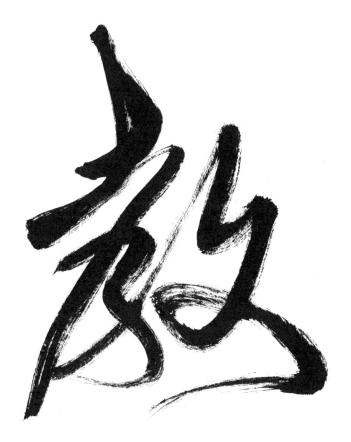

IN THE SPIRIT OF COACHING

Perhaps the two most important questions on this quest (quest-ions) that must be asked by all of us before we continue along this path are: First, why do you do what you do? This relates to the motivation underlying your work. Second, what is your purpose and intention? The answers to each of these deeply spiritual queries will serve as beacons or lighthouses on the horizon that will keep you on target. These questions require you to dig down deep inside and search for a higher purpose, one that ultimately relates to the spirituality of coaching.

My approach and assumption is that coaching is a human endeavor, one of creating healthy, enthusiastic, passionate athletes and teams. Athletes and coaches are spiritual in nature, have bodies, minds, hearts, and aspirations. We are all spiritual beings having an athletic experience, as opposed to athletes and coaches having a spiritual experience. The more I include the whole person in my coaching, the more effective, satisfied, and successful I am. Spirituality plays a significant role in my coaching effectiveness as I continue to help others transform their view of sports and its role in the full development of all who participate. It is this spirituality of coaching that enables me to inspire and empower those whom I lead. Oren Lyons, leader, caretaker, and faith keeper of the Native American Tradition and a member of the Onondaga Council of Chiefs, claims that you can't have effective leadership without spirituality. In the absence of spirituality, you have a one-dimensional approach which is called the absence of heart.

Highly effective coaches are dual-dimensional in their leadership. First, they incorporate the necessary Xs and Os, details, strategic planning, technical information, and other essential cognitive absolutes that cover the physical aspects of their sport. Then, dancing between these essentials (see introduction for more on this) is the inspiration, the empowerment, the caring, respect, positive regard, and most importantly, trust and compassion, all those affective spiritual elements of the heart. These coaches are leaders who, through strong relationships, manage to guide their athletes to "go the distance" and realize their full potential in sport. It is no different than guiding your children as a good parent. The ancient Taoist sage, Sun-Tzu, author of the classic book, *The Art of War*, reminds us how to get the most from others by leading with heart:

*"Regard your soldiers as your children, and they may
follow wherever you lead. Look upon them as your
beloved sons and they will stand by you until death."*

His message of the heart to all generals, heads of state, and other leaders is as relevant in today's world of coaching as it was when he wrote this classic over two thousand years ago. Of the two dimensions it is this spiritual heart-related dimension that this book addresses. I aim to demonstrate ways that we can be better able to make the connection and dance between both dimensions and begin to be more open, trusting, vulnerable, confident, and aware that we are part of a larger game, greater than the one we coach. With the spirituality of coaching as a guiding light for our leadership, athletics becomes a conduit for inner growth, change, and expansion for those we coach, helping them to experience something other than the ordinary. This is when we all live, play, coach, and compete in alignment with our hearts, the place where we do our very best to be the best we can be. It is a sacred space of greater meaning, higher performance, and value to all of our physical, mental, emotional, and spiritual needs and all that we aspire to be.

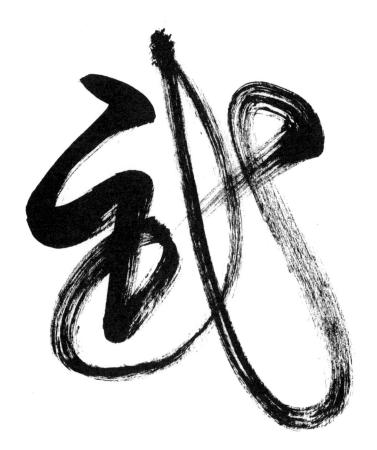

WU SHI LEADERSHIP

Ancient Chinese Taoist warriors were not interested in war, violence, and fighting to overcome others. They were heroic in nature, a culture of enlightened and awakened warriors possessing heart-felt traits and virtues. According to these great spirits, the power of these virtues was greater than the power of arms, the power one exerts over another in an authoritative way. Such evolved, cultivated, and civilized leaders were considered brave, compassionate, courageous athletes of iron will and indomitable spirit. They engaged in battles against fear, frustration, failure, and self-doubt while fighting for inner peace, strength, honor, majesty, love, gratefulness, trust, and respect. These battles were

fought with intangible weapons of the heart such as fearlessness, courage, patience, persistence, integrity, tenacity, and
fortitude. All obstacles were perceived as opportunities to
learn, grow, and become more aware of possibilities rather
than disabilities. In Chinese, this heart-felt spirit is referred
to as Wu Shi, the Warrior Spirit. It is a sacred spirit much in
alignment with the notion of the spirituality of coaching and
sports.

For practical purposes, I will define Wu Shi or the Warri-
or Spirit as a dance between striving to win, yet not needing
to win to be successful. It's a sacred space, one where you as
a coach embrace athletes as partners in a mentoring dance
of give and take, learning from each other what needs to be
known in order to advance and go the distance in sports
and life (see introduction for more). The Warrior Spirit
helps you to sacrifice and give to others, inspire them to
push past the breaking point, become comfortable with being uncomfortable, know when less is more, soft is strong,
accept responsibility, remain accountable, be willing to suffer, lose, be vulnerable, and fail if that's what it takes to ultimately win the battle before the war begins. The Warrior
Spirit, this "dancing heart of coaching" is all about being
mindful, self-aware, enthusiastic, passionate, spiritually and
emotionally alive, while providing safe environments that
help to cultivate peak capacities and potentialities through
the use and application of strong warrior heart-based virtues and behaviors.

The Taoist warrior leader relied heavily upon the wisdom
of the *Tao Te Ching*. Let me give you a glimpse of how this all
ties in with the spirituality, heart, and the love of coaching.

Basically, there is no need to go to a Taoist temple high in the mountains of China to be such a warrior leader. All you need to be is a good human being. Spiritual warriorship is not about mastering others but about mastering yourself.

And there is no path to such mastery: mastery is the path, an everyday practice of being kind, genuine, respectful, aware, vulnerable, balanced, humble, courageous, iron-willed, fearless, and intense yet calm. Traditionally, for such warrior leaders, war was a way of life. For the "new" warrior, life is a war, a battle of the inner struggles over self-doubt, fear, frustration, fatigue, and uncertainty. Armed with weapons of the heart, the warrior sees the bigger picture, thinks outside-the-box, trusts intuition, learns from failure, has pure intentions, acts with integrity, has passion, and love, and takes the higher road to do the right thing.

Very simply, as I state in the introduction to this book, with an increase of love, compassion, and spirituality in our coaching, athletes become happy, trust and respect deepen, and results and outcomes are significantly enhanced. When we develop Wu Shi (Warrior Spirit) relationships, those we lead are happy and work longer and stronger; when they work longer and stronger, results and outcomes usually improve.

The question we might ask is: how can you bring your full, complete, loving, human self to your coaching and use sports as a micro-cosmic classroom for personal, emotional, and spiritual growth for athletes and yourself in the arena of performance and in the bigger game of life? The answer, as we will discover, lies within the give and take dancing heart of Wu Shi leadership.

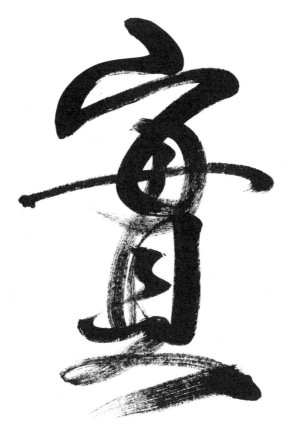

FIRMNESS YET FAIRNESS

With all the talk about kindness, caring, love, and heart, you may wonder if there's a place for being tough with your athletes, for raising your voice, for establishing strict boundaries, for using disciplinary measures. Absolutely, you can do all of this. In fact, if you really love your athletes, if you really care for them, to do anything less than this when appropriate would demonstrate a lack of caring. You are being kind when you enforce boundaries and refuse to tolerate a violation of team culture. Dancing heart coaches are very fair yet firm and these two items are not mutually exclusive.

He was one of the most fearless and highly respected

chiefs in the New York City Fire Department during his day. People under his command said how brave he was, leading dozens of men, half his age, into the belly of a raging fire. He led by example and guided others to places they needed to be. They listened to him because he was firm yet always fair. I learned my first lessons on leadership from this remarkable leader—he was my Dad.

The *I Ching*, the ancient Chinese book of change and transformation, validates what my dad intuitively knew to be correct. This *Tao* classic states that "it is necessary that a leader have firmness with fairness and an encouraging attitude toward others." Being strict yet impartial helps a leader to be admired, honored, and obeyed.

To be firm, you need to establish certain clear and understood boundaries, what will and will not be tolerated. The boundaries create a sense of security for your athletes. Knowing the parameters of behavior makes for clean, predictable, and familiar circumstances. Yet within these firm boundaries, there needs to be an element of fairness—treating others as they deserve to be treaded, with kindness and respect.

Coach John Wooden, of the UCLA basketball team, where he won 10 national championships, knows that being fair doesn't mean treating everyone alike. That's because everyone does not earn the same treatment. In his book *Wooden*, he explains that fairness is giving to others what they earn. He also points out that being fair at all times is not possible. He encourages making a sincere effort; others will recognize that about you, whether it's your kids, employees, or athletes. Wooden was respected by his athletes, and they competed and played with heart because he treated them firmly yet fairly.

To be fair in your leadership, you must refrain from making arbitrary decisions. For example, the star athlete is not given less of a punishment for wrongdoing than the athlete who hardly plays. Going outside the team boundaries—curfews, promptness, alcohol tolerance—calls for consistent consequences, regardless of one's role on the team. This is fair. And remember that with consistency of enforcement, there is order; inconsistent leadership leads to disorder. Along these lines, Sun-Tzu reminds us that if you show favor or indulge others, you are not coaching them well. That is not coaching with heart.

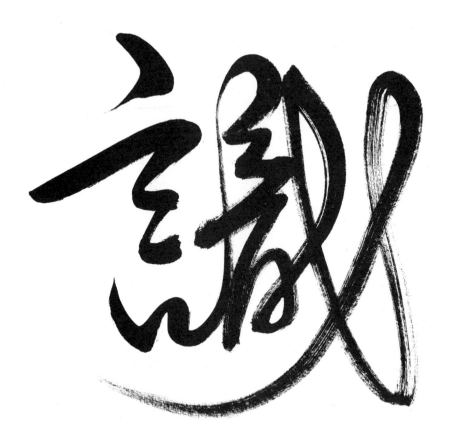

BEING THE FIVE SENSES

My work, at times, has not made sense. I have not made sense, as well. You want to be sure that your coaching style makes sense. Here are my Big 5, the five senses that make sense in order to be a sensible leader and coach…and sensitive as well.

1. A SENSE OF HUMOR. Hold yourself lightly. If you take yourself too seriously, you are in deep trouble. Your calling is serious business but not you. You are a silly, sometimes crazy, yet a great human and by definition you screw up, you fail, your athletes and followers fail, the Dali Lama fails…we are all human and this is how

it is. You are not your title, your position, your degrees, your possessions, or your status. At your core, you are simply a human being, and it would be a good act of compassion to accept yourself as such. I like to think about the leaders in the comedy series and movie, M.A.S.H. Who do you like and dislike? And why? Guess what? Those who had humor and didn't take themselves seriously were highly effective. You decide, but the role of humor in leadership and coaching is imperative for the "safe environment" we all wish to create. What you do is meaningful but that doesn't mean you must take it so seriously all the time.

2. A SENSE OF GENEROSITY. Think of coaching and leadership as a "giving process" not a "getting process." Look for ways to give, serve, and help. When a follower fails or does something wrong, give guidance, hope, caring, direction, forgiveness, and tolerance and watch them get quickly back on track. Be generous with love, respect, and trust. Care! You are a servant. More on service later.

3. A SENSE OF POSSIBILITY. Ask your followers to dream things that never were and ask, Why not? Promote courage to take risks and not worry about outcomes. The process of risk taking empowers them to keep going in the face of setback knowing that we all learn and improve in that way. No Risk, No Gain is my mantra.

4. A SENSE OF GRATITUDE. Help others to embrace what they have been given...healthy bodies, minds, hearts, opportunities, work, life. Have them understand that all successful people seem to have a deep sense of appreciation and their work and performance becomes a

huge reflection of that gratitude. I will go into greater detail with this as the book progresses.

5. A SENSE OF HUMILITY. Remember that we are all interconnected to something greater than self. I am quick to remind my seminarians and athletes whom I lead and coach that all of who I am and what I do is not my doing. Without others in my life—including those I lead and coach—I could not do what I do and would not be who I am.

I am honored and privileged to be asked by others to work with them.

They teach me all that I need to know so I can, in turn, teach them. It is a give and take and I humbly recognize and embrace that. It is the Wu Shi dance I wrote about earlier in this part of the book.

As I read over this Big 5, I realize that without these, I cannot do my work. My work is *being* these and from that place, my influence spreads…so will yours. When I disconnect from any one of these, I notice that I struggle in all of my life. I encourage you to practice these five in addition to all else that makes you shine.

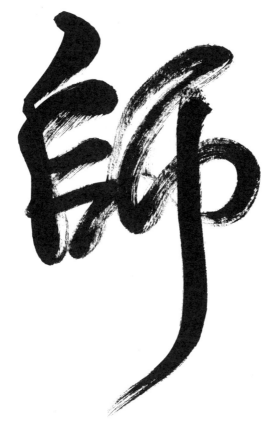

WHEN STUDENT IS READY,
TEACHER APPEARS

Do you ever wonder why you can't seem to motivate your athletes? How often do we as coaches and leaders become frustrated, upset, annoyed, perturbed, confused, puzzled, disgusted, perplexed, or completely baffled by our seeming inability to motivate and perform our task of coaching others? I can't begin to tell you how many times I have seen this happen. For example, I was talking with a coach recently who was concerned about three of his very talented athletes who were not listening and following his program. He was completely frustrated that he could not motivate these kids to raise their level of commitment to "go the distance" and realize their full potential. He was taking it very personally and was beginning to see himself as a failure. Truth is, bus drivers cannot transport others unless they get on the bus. (Have you noticed how often busses have the name "coach" written on the side? There is a reason for this). So it is as a leader and coach. The person must get on board with you (the bus) and be ready to travel to places they never dreamed possible. In Chinese there is a compelling expression that addresses this point: "When the student is ready, the teacher appears." Yes, and the teacher is usually there but without being ready, those followers are not aware of his or her presence.

Over the past 34 years of marinating my nervous system in the juices of leadership and coaching, what I notice is that no one can motivate others to move forward. You can inspire and empower them but they must want to move forward and when they do, the motivation comes from within. Change and growth is an extraordinary inner process and the work of a dancing heart leader is to be patient, persevere, and persist on nurturing and supporting, guiding and directing others in an environment that is emotionally safe from failure and taking risks. Your work as leader and coach is to add fuel to an already burning pilot light within your protégés. When you create a safe environment, you accelerate the process of readiness for others to be led. From this safe, sacred place, they will open their hearts to you and give you permission to enter. When you do, you will be able to do your best work. You will inspire, empower, and influence them to believe in themselves, to believe in you and to believe that they can be and do something other than ordinary.

If those you lead and coach are not moving forward, don't call 911 and don't try to motivate them, that is impossible to do. Instead, create a healthy relationship and environment that is emotionally safe (where failure is okay because it is our best teacher), listen to them, offer your help, and become the beacon that lights up the path. If they don't follow, keep trying, don't give up, don't ever give up and do not take it personally. Everyone has a different learning curve. And don't disregard the notion that following your path, what you think is best for everyone, may not be in their best interests. It's not about you, you're not a bad or inept coach. If you discover that they want out, if they want something different, are burned out, simply ask if they want you to release them to follow their hearts and discover what excites and energizes them. In another sense, to do such, to release them on another path is to be a very good coach. They will love you forever. I never witnessed a bus driver get off the bus and pull, shove, or coerce a pedestrian to get on board. But recently a driver asked me at the airport, "Are you getting on?" To which I replied, "No, thank you. I am waiting for someone to pick me up." Coaching is not much different. Ask those you lead: do you still want me to coach you, to bring you along? If they respond "no," then you might want to pursue this further. You want your athletes to be happy, to play for all the right reasons. It makes your life happier and easier.

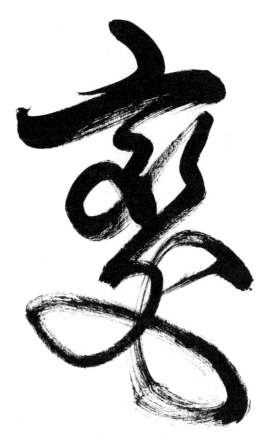

BE THE CHANGE YOU WANT TO SEE

When you drop a pebble in the center of a calm lake, the reaction created is a series of concentric circles that ripple across the water to the most distant shore touching everything in its wake. So it is with coaching and leadership. Who you are and what you do comes from your center, your essence, and as you talk, guide, mentor, and teach, your words and behavior ripple outward impacting and influencing all within your world. And that influence is never neutral; your body language, tone, words, habits, and behaviors will either light the fires of passion in those you coach and lead or douse their flames. (See Power of Influence in Part II.) To create growth and change in others, follow the advice of Gandhi who teaches us to be the change we want to see. In a word: *Model.* Model the behavior you expect others to emulate. I am always perplexed by coaches who demand fitness and wellness from their athletes and then proceed to stand on the sidelines chatting and laughing and watching as the athletes run, lift weights, and stretch their bodies to keep fit. What message does that send? When I coach a team, I always expect myself to do what I ask of them. I may not be as fit as them but I run, lift, and stretch with everyone. I recall when a nutrition expert was talking to a group of athletes and everyone was tuned out. At first I thought the athletes were being rude but the truth was, this "expert" was severely unhealthy and overweight. Why would they listen to him?

History tells us that in ancient times, the most respected generals did not seek comfort. They purposefully experienced the same adverse conditions—toil, hunger, thirst, cold—as their soldiers. They modeled what they expected from those they led.

Let the following questions help to guide you towards modeling what you want from those you lead:

1. How do you cope with failure?
2. How do you handle pressure and adversity?
3. How do you exhibit patience and persistence?
4. How do you create balance and congruity in your daily life?
5. How do you deal with criticism?
6. How do you listen?
7. How do you give to others?
8. How do you accept responsibility and be accountable for your actions?

9. How do you do all that you can to be the best you can be?

10. How do you show respect and trust in others?

How you express yourself with the above is how others will learn to express these items as well. You are the pebble and they are the recipients of its wake. Again, walk your talk. My rule of thumb when in leadership roles is: Never ask of others what you do not do yourself—or at the very least mimic in your own life on some scale. My favorite leadership/coaching story along these lines is about the time I was invited to give a keynote talk at the NIKE/China conference on Leadership. The day before my talk there was a 5K race with 135 participants from the conference…all of them athletic, senior executives with an average age of 30. I managed to win the race handily much to the surprise of this young group (they couldn't imagine this "older guy" being able to outrun them). I can tell you that I have never had such extraordinary attention at my presentation the following morning. They were ready to follow every word. I was able to use the race to my advantage. I led with my heart, legs, and passion and they seemed ready to follow wherever I went with the discussion, whatever I said.

Be the change you want to see.

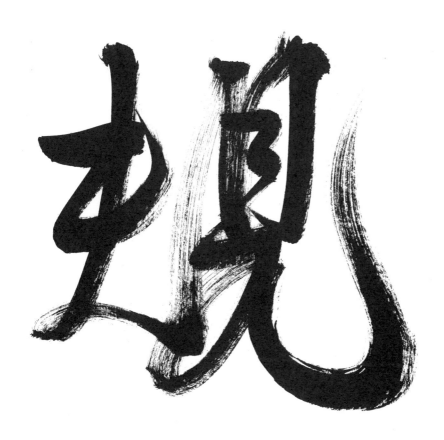

TEN EFFECTIVE BEHAVIORS

There are three secrets to effective leadership and coaching. Unfortunately, no one knows what they are. I have no secrets, but after years of being a leader/coach in some capacity, I have several observations that tell me what makes good leaders.

The following are a series of words and concepts that may be a good forum for discussion with your athletes, an opening to what it takes to be an effective coach and leader. All of these come under the umbrella of the most crucial behavior, which is the ability to be vulnerable.

1. Listener
2. Server
3. Trustful
4. Selfless
5. Flexible

6. Humorous
7. Compassionate
8. Humble
9. Respectful
10. Integrity

There are other behaviors, but without these, there is no leadership because there is no relationship and extraordinary leadership is only possible where strong positive relationships are formed, chiseled from the work of the heart.

I will promise you this: If you practice the above 10 behaviors, those you lead will follow you for a lifetime. How can you be good at being the above?

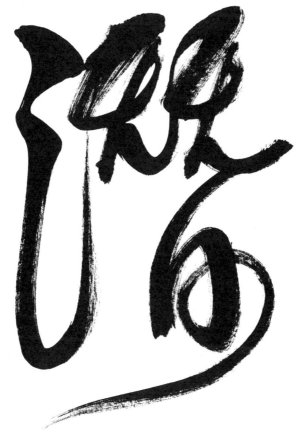

DORMANT LEADER WITHIN

I have observed that every one of us has the potential to be an extraordinary leader. In fact, I believe we are all good leaders yet for various interesting reasons, those innate, natural traits remain beneath the surface of our persona…in a word, they acquire the status of being Dormant—asleep, untapped, hidden—frozen in time only to be thawed when the need appears. For example, there is a story about some people standing around watching a young boy pinned under the wheel of a car that rolled down the driveway only to come to a stop on top of his little body. Amid the frantic crowd appears his 65-year old grandmother who lifts the car and directs the others to pull the boy from under the tire.

She demonstrated the leadership qualities of courage, determination, integrity, fearlessness, sacrifice, commitment, and audacity; traits she never believed existed within her.

Now, because I believe we all have wonderful leadership traits, I also believe that not all of us must or should be coaches. Even if you are considered by others to be a good coach, it's not a good enough reason to take on that role. You must have love and passion for wanting to serve others in this way—you must be eager and willing and ready to demonstrate those special qualities that we all have to different degrees. For those who choose not to take this path of coaching, that is perfectly fine, but know you choose so, not because you can't lead, but because you exercise your power of choice. Ironically enough, such a decision is, indeed, a leadership trait: you are a leader who coaches yourself to follow the path of your own heart.

Okay? Now, here is an exercise for you and your athletes to do. List 10 traits that you will find in good leaders you have known. Be brutally honest and underline 3 of those traits that you believe you have or are capable of demonstrating at various times. Now, if you have wanted to show leadership but have had the "I feel this is not me" syndrome, take those three traits and write down all the ways throughout the day that you can demonstrate these as a way to give and serve others from this place of leadership. Keep it simple, keep it specific, then proceed to watch how others respond to you and how you feel about exercising what were dormant traits. Only do this and be this way if you and your athletes have had the inkling to dabble with something new: simple, yet not easy. Yes?

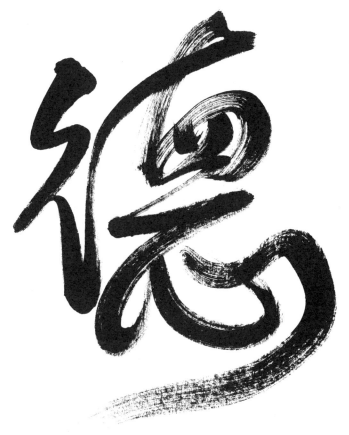

SOCRATES IN THE GYM

I refer to the word "power" not as exercising power over someone or something but the power to lead, guide, influence, inspire, and empower. In this sense, posing questions and their subsequent answers is a *Powerful* (full of power) way to guide others forward. The brilliant Greek philosopher, Socrates, taught in this fashion, using well thought-out questions to bring many of his followers' awareness on their journeys in life. After all, a journey is a *Quest for* wisdom and enlightenment and from the word "quest," we get "question," the means by which we discover the where, how, what, and why along the path. In my work, I am always using questions to help lead and coach others. I encourage them (give them courage) to search for the answers that ultimately reside within each of them. Later on in the book I will pose other questions that, when answered, will help to guide you as you guide those you coach.

The following are just the tip of the iceberg and I invite you to begin creating your own penetrating questions based on the needs and directions of athletes under your guidance. Have them write their responses and use that for lively discussion, learning, and awareness. And, let me suggest that you answer these questions yourself to help raise your level of leadership.

- What are the tangibles you bring to your group/team?
- What are the intangibles?
- What five things do you love about your sport/life?
- What are your personal goals for this next few months, what are the obstacles, how will you hurdle them? Be very specific giving measurable items.
- If you freed yourself to perform to your capacity, what do you imagine is possible?
- What are three ways that you can best serve your group/ team?
- What five specific behaviors/things can you do each day that will make you happy?
- What coach do you admire and why? What three behaviors define this individual and how can you begin to imitate these traits in your life?

Okay, you may want to steer clear of these next questions. Although I have personally found this one to be the most important and penetrating question one can ask in life, it can get pretty darn wild. And, it could require years to fully answer. Ready? Who am I (really)? Why do I do this work? How do I do it? Where am I going? Who do I wish to take with me? All great leaders and coaches have, in some way, answered these questions.

   You will notice how most, if not all, of these questions are internally focused and have a spiritual component. Remember that as a coach, your athletes' performance has much to do with body, mind, and spirit. That's why we all need to meet Socrates in the gym.

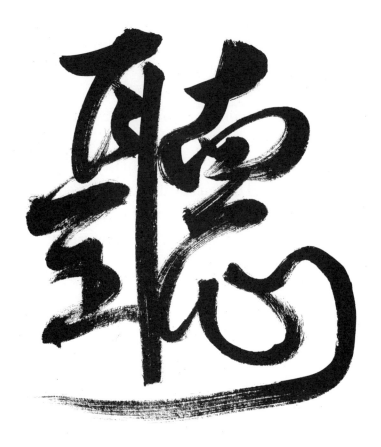

THE ART OF LISTENING

Wise leaders immerse with others refusing to
act judgmentally.
In this way, everyone opens ears, hearts, minds,
more able to understand the needs of others.

Tao Te Ching no. 49

It has been said that he who listens with an open heart, understands. The art of listening is one of the most crucial skills a coach can develop. Because so many of us feel that we need to talk in order to teach, listening is often overlooked. What I have observed over the years is that the very popular, well-liked coaches are, indeed, good listeners. Yet it has been observed that three out of four leaders and coaches will interrupt their staff and athletes on average, within 15 seconds of the start of a conversation. Such a practice precludes you from truly learning from others what you need to know in order to do your best work. How can you build a strong relationship in this way? How do you feel when those you lead listen to you? Could it be that they feel the same way when you listen to them?

Listening is an extraordinary way to demonstrate caring, respect, love, and integrity. Learning and teaching are more easily and joyfully exchanged through good listening as well. It is a way to make the athlete feel wanted, valued, worthwhile, and understood. Isn't this exactly what all coaches desire for their athletes? Those we lead feel the same way.

To develop the delicate art of listening, often referred to as unconditional positive regard, there are certain attitudes that a coach must display. First of all, you must be willing to take the time to hear what is to be said. You need to have the heart-set that makes you eager to help. When the athlete talks about his or her feelings, you must convey acceptance by listening with your heart as well as your ears. You don't have to agree with them but you must accept those feelings as spoken by a human being who trusts and respects you.

Rarely do any of us get the opportunity to learn listening skills. Yet, they are simple skills even though not easy to use. If you have a strong desire to include the art of listening in your repertoire of coaching abilities, the following tools of inquiry will help you to engage the athletes, improve your relationships, solve problems, make good decisions, and create environments that are safe and more productive.

If you want to empower, support, gain, and give respect

to your athletes, to find answers, solve problems, and make them feel that they count then use the following listening skills the next time you go one on one with an athlete.

1. DOOR OPENERS — a way to invite the other person to say more in a noncommittal way: "I see"; "Really"; "Interesting"; "Is that so?"; "You don't say"
2. STEPPING INSIDE THE DOOR — invitation for the other person to go further and be more explicit: "Tell me more"; "I'd like to hear about it"; "Let's discuss it"
3. KEEPING THE DOOR WIDE OPEN — this is infinitely the most effective of the three. You decode what the real message is:
   A. Try to understand what sender is feeling or means
   B. Put into your own words and feed back what you believe you hear; "It sounds like…"; "What I hear you saying…"; "Correct me if I'm wrong…"

For listening to be effective, give feedback for *only* what you feel is the sender's message, nothing more, nothing less. And do not warn, moralize, lecture, judge, blame, or criticize. With experience, you will grow more direct and intuitive; for now, simply use what another says and put it in your own words. At first it may feel contrived or awkward. That's okay; just do it anyway and tell others that it helps you to understand better.

These simple yet powerful skills will not just help your athletes to perform at higher levels, they will move them to a spirit of unparalleled loyalty and you will gain their compliance as you direct them into areas of greater development personally as well as athletically.

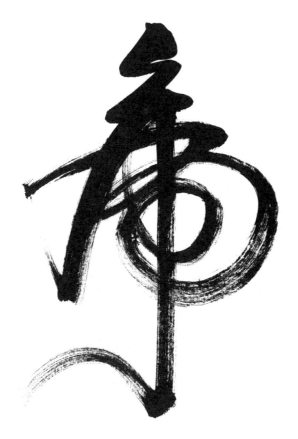

STRENGTH OF TEN TIGERS

I have been talking about the art of spiritual leadership and coaching with heart. I believe that it is imperative to not only grow our teams but to grow ourselves as well. As a coach, the self growing and expansion process is a spiritual exercise. You are a spiritual being having a leadership experience, not a leader having a spiritual experience. Leadership of any kind is first and foremost, a human endeavor. This human element in athletics and life is often sacrificed at any costs for "the bottom line": results, winning, and advancing. However, it is now known that the more attention we give to personal growth and development, the happier and more productive we will all be.

There is a way, an easy method to help facilitate such development. Some refer to this as the "Still Point." Most who practice this spiritual discipline use the term *Meditation*, a place of inner calm, clarity, peace, and quiet, and often gained (there are other ways) from focusing on a stationary object or watching the process of breathing. There is an ancient Taoist proverb that states: "If you know the art of breathing you have the strength of ten tigers." Over the years I have trained thousands of coaches and athletes in this skillful art using a 2500 year old form of Buddhist meditation called Vipassana, a Pali word that when translated means insight. This meditation practice relies on the awareness that breathing is happening and using the breath as a focal point to quiet what Buddhists call the "Monkey Mind." This meditative state of mind, this still point, is a sacred space that raises awareness, makes movement effortless, and confidence more robust. It helps us to find balance and keep it in our lives. It is a source of positive energy and keeps us connected to our purpose as coaches. While often seen as soft, weak, and intellectual, it has a direct positive influence on your overall effectiveness as a coach and, when practiced by you, your team, and athletes, contributes to higher more satisfying levels of performance. We must remember that between stimulus and response, there is a space. In that space you have the freedom and power to choose how you will respond to any given situation in the heat of battle or when positioned to make a problem solving decision. What meditation does is increase that space, improving the chances that the best will happen, that you will do the right thing and help you to identify, analyze, and understand essential issues in life. Metaphorically, you become like a high mountain lake on a windy day; your surface may be choppy but underneath the surface, there is a calmness of confidence that helps you to navigate the rough, turbulent waters. From this sacred state of mind, you develop a sense of peace and happiness that contributes extensively to coaching with heart. In this mindset you can find answers to the penetrating questions: Why do I coach? Why do I coach the way I do? How does it feel to be coached by me?

Not many know that former Hall of Fame coach of the world champion Chicago Bulls and Los Angeles Lakers, Phil Jackson, created what he called the "warrior room," a place where athletes were invited to come and meditate prior to a game. He found that this breathing practice helped his champions connect more strongly to the team's mission and goals.

In my work with highly functional collegiate and professional athletic teams and coaches, I train them to use meditation prior to practice and games. This helps them to get more out of their practice sessions and be more centered and focused on executing the game plan more effectively. This consistent practice of mindful meditation is exactly what was used by the Taoist warrior who sought to "settle" his mind for what became an undisturbed performance. It helped him to fight the inner wars of self-doubt, fear, and low confidence by focusing strictly on what he could control, all the little things, the essential absolutes of his craft. When this happens, confidence rises like a hot air balloon and self-doubt evaporates like moisture in a desert.

In my meditation practice, I rise each day and sit in quiet meditation for 20 minutes. I then visualize by *feeling* myself perform, compete, act, speak, work, socialize—basically a rehearsal of my day exactly the way I would like it to evolve. After about three or four minutes of this, I recite strong, short, positive, present-tense statements that affirm the direction I want my day, performance, and life to go. I finish each session by reminding myself of all that I am grateful for in this life—family, friends, home, food, work, health, and more—and tell myself to make the rest of the day—how I act, behave, and perform—a strong reflection of all that I have been given. (More about this later.) Taking the time to do this helps me to choreograph a highly functional and extremely happy and productive life.

If you want to find your "still point" try the following westernized meditative steps, a combination of Buddhist Vipassana Insight meditation, yoga breathing, and imagery psychology. With eyes closed, in a quiet place, free from interference, sit comfortably in a chair with back straight and feet on the floor. Drop arms into your lap:

1. BEGIN BY taking three deep, controlled breaths, holding the oxygen in your lungs for three seconds before you exhale. Notice how this procedure has an instant effect on your body and mind, relaxing you immediately. Then, stop and return to normal breathing.

2. SIMPLY NOTICE that breathing is happening. Watch it come in and go out. Do not control its natural flow other than to have it go through the nostrils.

3. WHEN YOUR mind wanders—and it will—simply acknowledge it and direct it back by saying "wandering, come back." Don't be concerned about the wandering: it's natural. In fact, the act of being aware of the

wandering and bringing your attention back to the breath, actually helps you to develop strong attention skills when performing, coaching, or competing in everyday life. It develops what we call Meta attention. Wandering is an integral aspect to the full meditation practice.

4. Do THIS "breath watching" for about eight minutes, then switch gears and begin to visualize by feeling yourself being how you wish to be at work, performing, coaching, competing, parenting, writing…whatever it is that you do. Visualize for about four minutes.

5. FOLLOWING YOUR visualization, recite a few short, positive affirmations that nurture and support your visualizations. Unlike visualizations which involve how you feel and what you see, these strong statements influence what you say and, more importantly, how you think. Thoughts strengthen or weaken you and determine the direction in which you go. Affirmations are spiritual gems that keep you on the path to coach with heart. Write them out on index cards and as you recite them, feel the words as if they are real and happening now.

Remember this: meditation practice is like physical training; it is exercise for the mind. Such exercise helps you to develop greater emotional intelligence. Well conducted scientific studies have demonstrated that after only eight weeks of meditation practice, the participants experienced much lower levels of anxiety, significant rise in positive emotions, and were measurably happier. As we know, focused, happy coaches and athletes are mentally tougher and experience higher levels of performance. There is an Asian saying that supplements these findings. It says that "the quiet, focused mind can pierce through stone." That's the strength of ten tigers.

Part One:
Wisdom to
Inspire

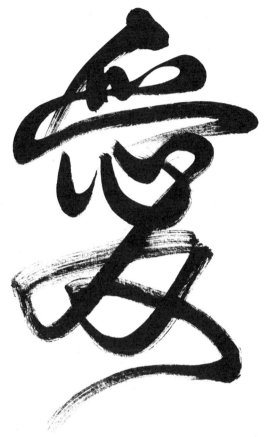

HAVING LOVE IN YOUR HEART

There is one language everyone understands throughout the world. It improves life, work, and performance. It is the language of love.

The element of love in coaching circles is so vital and crucial that I considered writing a whole book on this subject alone. I would have titled it: *For the Love of Coaching*. Actually, as you peruse each segment of this book, you will quickly observe and feel the interconnectedness of all topics with this notion of love. Mother Teresa's words on the importance of love speak volumes: "When we come face to face with God, we are going to be judged on how much we loved." So it is with coaching. When all is said and done, in retirement your career success will be measured by how much you loved. If you aspire to be an extraordinary coach, you must have love in your heart…no love, no coaching.

John Wooden, upon his retirement from basketball at UCLA, was asked by the media why he was so successful. His reply was: "It is simple; there was a lot of love in my coaching."

Grambling State football coach, Eddie Robinson, after he replaced coach Bear Bryant atop footballs' wins list, said the secret to his success was love. "Coaching is a profession of love. You can't coach athletes unless you love them." Loving athletes, in fact, will inspire and empower them to go the distance.

Perhaps underlying most difficulties athletes have with coaches is the deep longing we all have to be loved, cared for, respected, and cherished. According to the teachings of the Chinese sage Confucius, "when the ruler cherishes affection and love for his kindred, there will be no disaffection among members of his family." The best leaders really do care about those under their guidance. Military books are replete with stories of how the best of officers loved and cared for those under their command.

Coach Dean Smith is an example of a loving coach. In his book, *The Carolina Way*, he mentions that "I truly cared about what happened to our players at Carolina while in school and after they graduated. I became close to them." It was love that was central to the athlete-coach relationship at Carolina.

The *I Ching* makes it clear that warrior Taoist leaders must nourish, support, and love those led, in order to create unity and power within the group. Sun-Tzu, in his *Art of War* alludes to the importance of generals loving and taking care of the troops as one would take care of a child who was loved.

By so doing, the chances for victory in all their endeavors was greatly enhanced.

Love has many far reaching effects on the athletes under your heart-filled guidance. Let me explain what I mean. Most coaches crave mental toughness in their athletes. You don't win tough games with talent. You win tough games by being tough and that toughness comes when there is love. When athletes feel safe, respected, and loved they will go the distance, all out, relentlessly, so darn mentally tough that they begin to annoy their opponent. They become a huge pest. I believe we all do under the right environment of love. And, remember, athletes often give up when tired, but with love, they are tenacious even if totally fatigued. With an environment of love modeled by the coach, athletes will always battle and fight to the death for something bigger than just winning, something greater than themselves. This was demonstrated in extraordinary fashion by the coaches and athletes of the 2013 woman's lacrosse National Champions at the University of North Carolina. They were exhuasted in triple overtime yet never caved in because of the relentless love from the staff and athletes for each other. They fought for something greater than themselves as they won their first championship.

In addition to this toughness factor, environments where love proliferates are filled with discipline. When athletes have love, they refuse to let their team and staff down and this is what creates discipline in such caring and loving environments.

Now, how do you, as a coach with heart, demonstrate this intangible yet "feeling" concept of love? I have many ideas that stand the test of time. For example, attend to the deep-ness of commitment. By this I mean nurture the commitment athletes have to each other. Encourage the commitment between coaches themselves. And remember the commitment between coach and athlete and vice versa. Such commitment is nurtured and strengthened by giving: giving to others, giving your trust, respect, selflessness, integrity, and work ethic. Giving through hard work is, in my opinion, one of the more powerful expressions of love. Work is love made visible. So we have love which brings about giving that leads to commitment. According to the late charismatic leader Martin Luther King Jr., the most important question one can ask in life is: "What am I doing for others?" How can I give versus how can I get is a nice focusing statement to keep you and your athletes on track. And remember this universal truth: you may think you have a lot in life, but if you are without love, you have nothing.

To demonstrate a coach's traits of love and caring, I also suggest that you try my "rule of one": one athlete, one positive comment, and one day at a time. Of course when you do this, it becomes contagious and you won't be able to stop, like any habit. And you will see the results. You may say: "Hey, Britt, I love the way you show up ready to play each practice. You really set a terrific tone for this team." That will stay in her heart for at least three weeks when it will be time to begin again.

My favorite story using the "rule of one" is about an assistant coach who was struggling with a very good athlete with a very poor attitude. Jenn was catching this athlete doing the wrong things at practice and this athlete was being somewhat rebellious over the coach's criticisms. I suggested to Jenn that she use the "rule of one" and try to catch the athlete doing something right and reward her for it. I make a huge effort to be quick to find praise yet slow to find fault. Two weeks later, she told me her athlete had a major turnaround. Their relationship became a joy to watch. On Jenn's birthday, as she entered her office to begin the day, she was greeted with the most beautiful bouquet of flowers with a note from this athlete expressing her gratitude for Jenn's new approach. I witness life's changes like this often, the result of the "rule of one" where we demonstrate the ability to arouse enthusiasm, encouragement, excitement, gratitude, and appreciation in others. These are the greatest skills and assets one can possess.

Another way to demonstrate caring is to send an email or leave a note in a locker telling another how in awe you are of him or her. Tell the group/team how fortunate you are to be a part of their amazing lives. But most of all, always, every day, hour, minute, treat those you lead with respect and kindness and take good care of them. Be firm and set boundaries where and when needed but always do it in the spirit of the warrior, just the same way that you love to be loved. When that happens, others will follow you to the ends of the earth.

Then, there are those moments in life when you must critique an athlete on his or her performance. To do so in a loving, caring fashion, try the PCP method: *Positive* opening, direct *Critique*, *Positive* close. For example, you may say something like: "Hey, Chip, I love the way you come to practice ready to play. That shows good leadership on your part. Now, if you want to take it up a notch, try communicating more often while you're practicing, getting your team to follow your directions. That's better leadership. Want you to

know that you are an important part of our lacrosse family."
How would you feel after such an interaction with your
coach?

In her best-selling book, *A Return to Love*, Marianne Wil-
liamson talks about the power of love to empower others to
grow, expand, and develop personal potential. According to
her, love is a topic that must be taken seriously if positive
change is to take place. She believes that miracles happen
when we make love the bottom line in our environments
and relationships. As a coach, love is my bottom line. I seek
multiple ways to remove all the barriers to love such as fear,
self doubt, and uncertainty, and watch the miracles occur as
a natural expression of that love.

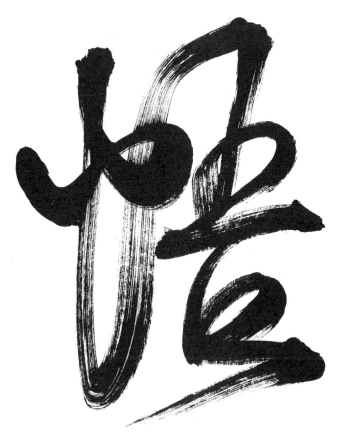

GUIDING IN SACRED AWE

Here is what I believe to be a highly effective guide and extraordinary affirmation for any of us who wish to coach with love, one that if taken to heart, will change your leadership style and the lives of those whom you lead in a remarkable and inspiring way. It sums up everything I've been saying about having love in your coaching. It is something I wrote after reading a statement by Rudolph Steiner, on his philosophy of teaching in the Waldorf school system. Place it on a placard and hang it in your office as a daily affirmation that you coach with heart.

Regard those you lead in sacred awe;
Coach and serve them in love.
Cultivate and teach in an envrionemnt of heart,
And watch as they grow into
Something extraordinary.

Remember this: when you treat athletes as they ought to be, not as they are, they become so much more.

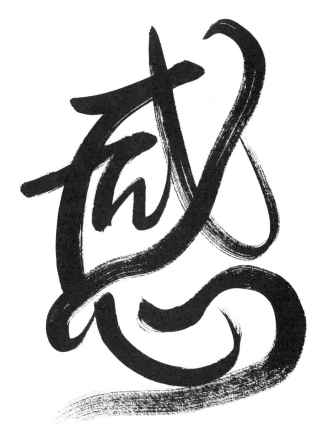

GRATEFUL TO GREAT

Tao means the Way, the way things are. It is a way to practice celebrating the present as you become conscious of what is genuinely important. The dancing heart coach takes nothing for granted. Such coaching is about acknowledging the gifts of life and holding the feeling of gratitude deep within so that you can coach with a clear mind and a focused heart. In the beginning of this book you read about how, as coaches, we are blessed. The awareness of this originates deep within our sense of gratefulness.

Gratitude is the extraordinary appreciation for one's blessings. Being grateful contributes to overall good health and well-being and fosters stronger relationships. It helps you to manage stress, lowers the rate of depression, and contributes to overall happiness. Shared gratitude, I can anecdotally report, between coaches and athletes, is emotionally satisfying, promotes a stronger sense of team, and has a strong, positive effect on performance. Basically, it is a process of going from grateful to great.

The process of developing a *Tao* of Gratefulness, modifying our thinking to entertain positive thoughts, is completely within our control. It means developing a habit, a practice, like anything else worthwhile. All successful coaches whom I admire have this "attitude of gratitude." For me, it is complete joy working with them. Think about how it feels to be around ungrateful, entitled people. This is exactly how athletes feel being coached by ungrateful leaders.

I often conduct the following exercise on gratefulness with my teams prior to an important practice or a game that needs to be played with high-level intensity and integrity.

Before they begin their workout, training session, or work for the day, I ask coaches and athletes to think of seven aspects of life that they appreciate. For example, their skills, talents, mind, health, family, opportunities, and work. Now, with eyes closed, I ask that they connect to the feeling of gratefulness. I tell them to imagine this feeling and take it into the body in three deep breaths, as each breath surrounds the heart. Hold each breath there as the feeling begins to expand. With this sensation of gratitude in the heart, I ask that they make their performance today a reflection and extension of that appreciation.

Now, they open their eyes and take on the day's tasks. I say to them, if you are grateful and appreciative of your health, feel your vitality. If you are appreciative of your talents, be sure to use them consciously this day. If you have a great family, be certain you communicate your love, caring, and gratitude to them. I then ask them to notice the difference in how they perform. Such ordinary moments create the extraordinary in all you do.

Often times I personally experience this exercise following my meditation practice. I love to remind myself of the importance of giving back to others through my work for all that I have been given in my life at this moment. This could help you, as well, in your coaching each day before you go to work.

Another gratefulness exercise I use in my coaching is to have my team sit in a circle and ask them to tell the teammate to their left what they appreciate about them as a person and as a significant athlete on the team. The room becomes inundated with love as the bond between them gets even stronger. This works especially well prior to a big tournament or at another significant time during the season.

Finally, I love to write a daily email of gratitude to a friend or colleague, or athlete, to help set a positive tone not only for them but for myself as well. When you give love you get it back a hundred times. When I do this, I feel more optimistic, more alive, and better about my life. It has been scientifically shown that such gratefulness increases the activity in the brain's pleasure centers. And who of us does not enjoy pleasure?

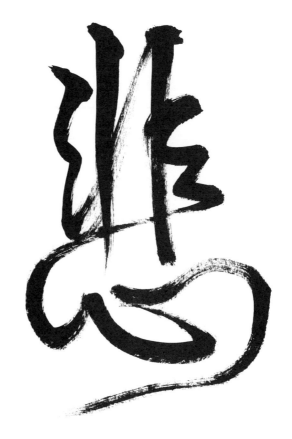

THE LENS OF COMPASSION

*Leaders whose positions endure are those who are
the most compassionate; when two armies meet,
the one with compassion is the one that tastes victory.*

Lao-Tzu

Associating with extraordinary coaches over the years has taught me the importance of compassion in all aspects of life. Personally, I consider it one of the more important essential absolutes for effective, heart-directed leadership. It is a state of happiness that requires emotional intelligence and engagement with those you lead. It is a state of heart and mind for the concern of others, a "we" versus "I" approach to life. In athletics, this translates into one's willingness to coach, compete, play, and work with an open heart, being compassionate toward yourself, your athletes, staff, friends, coworkers, and opponents. Compassion is seeing life through a different lens—in some cases, through others' eyes. It is a form of love and empathy that helps improve performance and fuels the fire of the heart as it unites teams; as former coach Phil Jackson claims, it was compassion that allowed his world champion Chicago Bulls to sustain high levels of excellence.

According to the *Tao Te Ching*, compassion ignites the courage within, giving one a sense of comfort and security in knowing that when risks are taken, regardless of the outcome, you will be fine. Knowing that compassion is available, you essentially have permission to fail, not that you would choose such an outcome. You gain, with compassion, the safe inner and outer environments that encourage ("instills courage in") you to trust in yourself, your team, coworkers, family, and friends and to continue to try again and again in the face of adversity. When, as a coach, you model such heart-directed behavior, you influence all who come under your guidance and direction.

Because of compassion, courage is able to flourish in such safe environments. The word courage comes from the French word *Coeur*, meaning "heart." Courage allows you to coach and perform with heart, to be brave, fearless, tenacious, and relentless. This is contagious with your athletes as well. You become more courageous when you know that compassion is available if you fail, make a mistake, or lose.

Adhere to the Zen Buddhist expression "The arrow that hits the bull's eye is the result of one hundred misses." As a performer in other arenas of life, it's compassion that helps you to take risks and keep shooting the arrows when failure, setbacks, and mistakes are experienced on the journey. Courage becomes compassions' strong emotional and spiritual partner, which helps you to realize that you have nothing to lose and everything to gain.

Think about what your world would be like if you treated others and yourself with love and compassion. Get "inside the skin" of your athletes and try to understand their situation without judgment. Enter the internal world of your athletes. Help them to feel understood and accepted. This basic value of coaching helps you to help athletes to "go the distance." It's what many refer to as being emphatic. The word "compassion" literally means to "suffer with." Understand, too, that you and those athletes are part of something larger than yourselves, and setbacks are part of the process of learning to get better. As we know, failure is an invaluable teacher. I notice how my ten greatest successes in life are the result of a thousand setbacks, mistakes, and failures. Great teams surge ahead of the pack following devastating defeats because they have marinated their nervous systems in a culture of compassion and courage.

This natural, softer yet stronger approach to sport and other arenas of performance and competition helps you to be more tolerant and accept failure in yourself and others, which, interestingly enough enables you to go forward in the exploration of you and your athletes' vast potential. Remember, there are only two kinds of athletes and coaches in the world: those who fail, make mistakes, and commit errors and those who will. Repeat this affirmation often: "Rather than be judgmental and critical of self and others, I choose to put my heart on the line and act with courage and compassion."

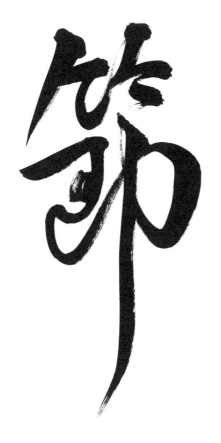

CYCLE OF FOUR SEASONS

Part of your mission of coaching with a dancing heart is to teach your athletes to take responsibility and accountability for what they do. What better time to do this than during what we traditionally refer to as the "off season." In college athletics, this occurs during the three month period called summer. Other sports and situations may have varying off seasons so they can adjust accordingly. I'll leave that in your hands. But the concept holds for everyone. I call this fourth season, the *Investment Season*. It is one of the four seasons during a calendar year. In China, the cycle of four seasons defines a complete experience creating lasting good and positive change in habits and ways. I've adapted this idea to athletics, to have four distinct, forward moving seasons, a complete experience creating sustained, consistent, higher levels of growth and improvement.

The length of each season will vary with each sport. All are approximately three months in duration; some are longer than others. For example basketball, baseball, football, and lacrosse can be four or more months. In college, cross-country and track are a full nine months. But my point is to get athletes to accept responsibility and accountability for the time when they are not physically present "on campus" during the school year. Aside from the *Investment Season* (and I will explain this in a moment), we have the conditioning, skill work, and mental mechanics season, the spring and fall ball seasons (out of season play) and the in-season season. The traditional "off season" usually comes between November 15th and February 15th or sometime during the summer vacation.

The *Investment Season* is a time where athletes commit to investing in self and team in order to maintain fitness, gain the competitive advantage over other teams, and to give back to the team. No one will be watching so it demands a high level of integrity and deep sense of intention, purpose, and commitment. The overall goal is to position oneself for having an extraordinary in-season by investing, giving, and contributing out of caring and love for each other. Such an investment is made so as to reap the dividends from all your hard work down the road. Here are a few questions that should help direct your athletes to make significant investments in their program and team. By the way, this is also valuable for the coaching staff to do and therefore, be good role models for the athletes. Answer the following and be brutally honest:

1. What specifically do you need to do in order to show up on (fill in the date) at a higher level than you are now?
2. Which of these listed tasks are you eager to realistically commit to as an investment in yourself and your team?

Once the athletes have their answers completed, sign the commitment sheet, combine everyone's investment, and make sure each athlete has a complete packet that includes all team members and staff. This last part accomplishes two things: it could help other athletes in the group to expand their list by discovering things to do they didn't know could be done and it could also help to recruit other training buddies who wish to accomplish similar things. Also, they can email or text each other to see how progress is going. This will keep the motivation alive and well between them. The power in this exercise is in each athlete's willingness to design a program, take responsibility, and be accountable to themselves and teammates. As their coach, you do not need to get involved other than to occasionally ask how it is going and if anyone needs help.

Remind the team of this fact: champions do what others are not willing to do. Champions do the right thing—especially when others are not looking.

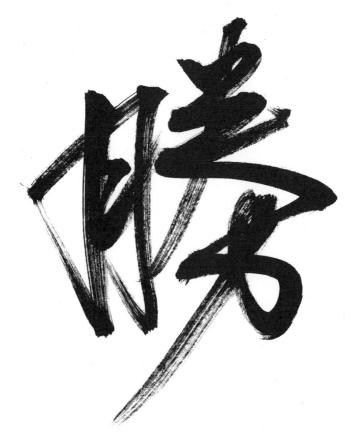

INVICTUS SPIRITUS

On his deathbed, Napoleon Bonaparte uttered the words: "…the sword is always beaten by the spirit." The spirit cannot be defeated unless you succumb. In Latin, the words *Invictus Spiritus* translated mean the undefeated spirit. You may defeat me on the scoreboard but I will refuse to let you defeat my spirit, my heart, soul, what I am, who I am, what I can do, and how I do it. When I battle with my heart, for the love of competing, and go the distance, my performance, win or lose, is uncategorically brilliant. I can control this and have confidence in my ability to do so. The outcome will take care of itself. This paragraph needs to be read to your athletes several times.

As a coach, you can develop a culture where your athletes prepare, play, and perform with heart (see section: "Culture of We Not Me"). And this requires their commitment to developing great spiritual strength through your guidance and leadership. World Champion runner, Herb Elliott, undefeated in competition, once said "I came to realize that enormous spiritual strength had to be stored up before a race." A huge part of my work with coaches is to help them to help their teams build up massive reservoirs of spiritual strength to enable them to compete with heart.

One of these teams is the University of North Carolina women's lacrosse program that I have previously mentioned. For the past three consecutive years we have been competing in the Final Four wearing a shirt that said across the chest, "INVICTUS SPIRITUS." As I have already mentioned, we have just won our first national championship with the undefeated spirit as our mantra. These warrior athletes had a deep commitment, dedication, and resolve to never, ever give up, to give their all, go the distance, and demonstrate the heart of the champion. Their head coach, Jenny Levy, has a spirit that is *Invictus* (and infectious by the way) in nature. She is an extraordinary model of what she expects from her "kids." Such attitudes are taught and bred in her culture of champions, a team with heart who play their very best to be the best they can be. Their confidence comes from knowing that regardless of who they play, they may lose on the scoreboard but the opponent will never defeat their spirits; they win the battles of the heart against inner fear, frustration, fatigue, and self-doubt. Their rewards are deeply personal and satisfying. They believe in themselves and display strong, consistent efforts to do all that it takes to get it done. When they lose, they are disappointed yet embrace the setback as a teacher, learn, and forge ahead. They are heart-directed athletes: tenacious, fearless, proud,

and confident to be Invictus in all they choose to do. They fully grasp the difference between what they can control (their spirits) and cannot (outcomes and results) and choose to focus on the former. For them, with *Invictus Spiritus*, winning becomes a multidimensional experience of inner victory, demonstrating personal greatness, and, hopefully, achieving favorable outcomes as well. This is a Tao, a way, to navigate the journey of infinite potential, assured that you will discover how great you can be, capable of reaching extraordinary levels of personal best performance. This way is a choice and all your athletes have the power to choose to be the Invictus Spiritus, the extraordinary, champion way.

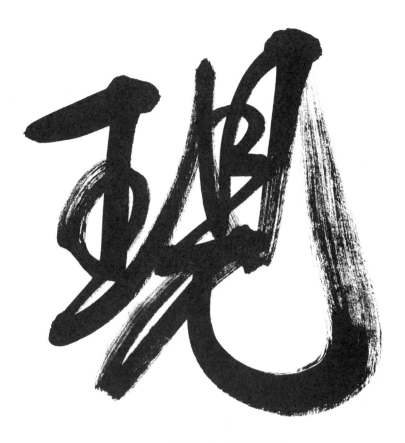

BE HERE NOW

It is always a good idea to be aware of when we are following a script in life whether we are coaching, teaching, presenting a talk, leading, acting, or playing an athletic game. We follow what's written on sheets of paper or what we think is expected from us by others (peers, audiences, fans, coaches, and teachers) in position to judge and criticize what we do. We fear that we may forget what's to be said, fear that we will make a mistake, look silly or foolish, look unprofessional, ignorant, unknowing, and basically, afraid to be open, vulnerable, transparent, and authentic.

Unfortunately, following the script blindly is a sure way to get yourself in trouble and not be present in the moment.

I find that the more I rely on the script, the further I separate myself from my heart, my passion, and the deep connection I wish to have with others. Yes, I do perform, and that is important, but "doing a performance" needs to be accompanied by "being": being genuine, authentic, transparent, present, focused in the now, and confident in simply executing the little things that make big things happen (from little streams come big rivers). My performance is not about strategies, techniques, power points, skill demonstration, information dissemination…it's about being present and trusting what I have within—knowledge, wisdom, innate and emotional intelligence—and allowing it all to flow in an environment that is internally and externally emotionally engaging and safe from criticism and failure. Your impulse may be in the realm of doing rather than in the realm of being. It's who you are being that will determine the depth, quality, and importance of relationships, and your followers' eagerness to be loyal, respectful, and attentive to your wishes. As Ram Dass says in his book by the same title: *Be Here Now.*

What I want to continue to practice—and I have practiced this for 34 years now—is to be present: *how can I* be present, genuine, and focused on the little things. It is then, and only then, that I can have my greatest influence in bringing truth, joy, empowerment, and inspiration to those willing to open their hearts to such an experience. This is simple, *but* not easy to do while coaching with heart.

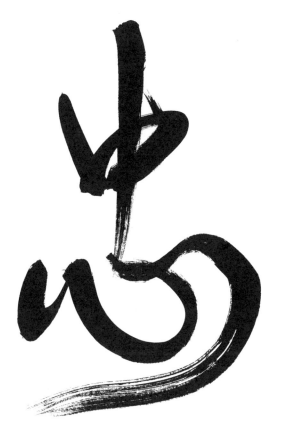

ONE HEART, ONE GOAL

Over many years of conducting team building sessions with champions, I find that the more I offer the athletes an opportunity to unite, come together, and create a oneness of heart, oneness of goal, the commitment to the team imperative becomes stronger. This process is very much like what we can observe during murmuration, as flocks of thousands of starlings fly through the air in Tai Ji fashion, one movement, one heart, one goal—as if a single soul.

What I am basically communicating to my teams is the importance of uniting our hearts, both staff and athletes, with one common thread that makes it clear: *It's all about*

US, and the "US" piece stands for *United Spirits* in a cohesive whole committed to doing all that we can to be the best we can be, on and off the field. This becomes our mission statement with the goal of positioning ourselves for winning on the scoreboard and possibly the national championship.

United Spirits have no need to worry about their opponents. This is because they commit to competing with heart for a goal well beyond merely beating others. It is a goal to play for a higher purpose, for the love, caring, and respect for each other. Such a goal inspires all of us to work harder and smarter. Because we fight and battle for those we love, we are relentless, never back down, and put forth all we have left in the tank. Our confidence rises because we believe these are things we can control as opposed to beating others, an uncontrollable and tension producing venture at best. When you focus in on outcomes and results and awards, you become tight, tense, and tentative thus creating sub-par performance, lowering confidence, and raising self-doubt. The confidence of *United Spirits* is rooted in the knowledge that they have done all that they could to prepare themselves to battle at the highest level. Their opponent may perform at higher levels but united spirits simply concentrate on being US, United Spirits. It's all about US. It says that we love the struggle, the fight, the suffering. We keep the goal of winning in our heads but know that the battle itself is in our hearts. As Sun-Tzu says in *The Art of War*, the war is won before the battle begins because of US.

All of what I have just described was demonstrated recently when the University of North Carolina women's lacrosse team won their first national championship following five years of developing the "one heart, one goal" culture, committing to competing as one heart, one soul. They played not to win the championship, but for something higher, for each other, for their love of the game, and winning the inner heart battles. Here is an excerpt from and email sent to me from the coach, Jenny Levy, following the victory: "It was the most amazing game I've ever been a part of... the spiritual side of the game was astounding. They fought together as one, with poise and belief. They never gave up into triple overtime. We won a championship, yes, but it was something bigger, more than a trophy. We learned lessons for life. The grit, courage, resilience, fearlessness, and toughness will never be forgotten. It is now in the fabric of who we are." This is what all of my teams feel when they compete with heart, with soul, one spirit, one goal.

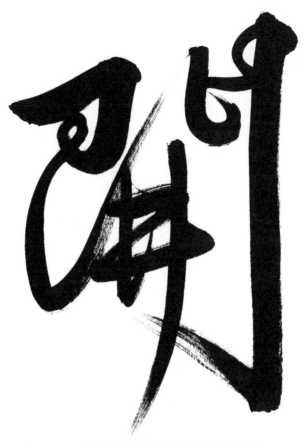

OUTSIDE-THE-BOX

When you first arrive at the home page of my website (www.wayofchampions.com) you quickly become aware of the fluid movement of my provocative Chinese logo. But, if you look closely, are you aware of the dancing hearted warrior coach, leader, athlete in the middle of the red box breaking free from the confines, throwing arms and legs to the outside? Notice how the color of this figure changes from black to a shade of gray? Let me explain the subtle shifts going on before your eyes. The Warrior is trapped inside the box where everything is black and white (the colors literally are black and white), right or wrong, good or bad, winner or loser. The Warrior knows that such dualities must be neutralized if success is to be attained. For example, loss isn't good or bad; it's a teacher helping us to refine our game and learn then move forward. Also, our opponents aren't the bad guys; they are partners who, because of their presence, challenge us to improve and bring out our best. Sometimes, less is more and soft is strong (water is soft but wears away rock). Such thinking is counter-intuitive for most of us but for the dancing heart coach there is no other way: we must break out and transform. But it takes sacrifice, suffering, and pain to change, to be different, and to follow your heart and not the orders of the masses. That's why the box is symbolically colored red, the Chinese color for fire (pain, suffering) change, and transformation. Anything that comes in contact with fire is changed and transformed. Notice the warrior goes from black to a shade of gray when exiting the red box. Red is also the color of heart and passion, meaning in this case, follow your heart and what you love, and all will work out the way it is supposed to.

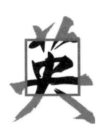

So what is the importance of this, and what significance does it have in the work of coaching with heart? Only you can answer this question for yourself. However, I have noticed that extraordinarily heart-directed, successful coaches seem to have a way of living outside-the-box. They are unusually inspirational and empower others to seek their individual and collective greatness. By reading this book on coaching, you are obviously aware of how much of the material is different from the norm; rather it is filled with unconventional and refreshingly stimulating outside-the-box thinking. By looking at my Warrior Logo, I am constantly reminded about the importance of such thoughts while it keeps me focused on what matters. This is the way, the *Tao*, of the dancing heart coach.

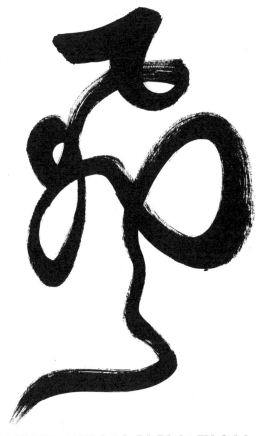

INSPIRATION ELEVATION

Inspiration is one of those intangibles that most of us crave, but very few are able to access when needed. You may shout to your athletes "Get inspired!" or "Play Inspired!" yet nothing seems to happen without some touchstone or reference point.

First off, it's important to know that, by definition, inspiration refers to any stimulus that causes creative thought or action. Elevating your spirit requires a prompting from something perceived, written, or said, or the presence of a particular person or object, all of which gives life or courage at work or in the heat of performance. Being inspired helps you to become more focused, animated, and motivated to carry out a desired task.

My experience shows me that many top athletes elevate their spirits with a simple act of consciousness. They may think about a song, a poem, a passage from a book— like the *Bible*, *Koran*, or *I Ching*— a friend, a parent, a character in a movie, or even someone they do not know but have heard about such as the Dalai Lama. You, as their inspirational coach, can help them to be inspired by posting words, thoughts, or ideas on their locker doors or by simply texting or emailing them at an appropriate moment, words that encourage, empower, inspire, and influence.

When you are coaching on the court or field, or in the locker room, getting ready to give a pre-game talk or simply helping an athlete on the sidelines, and you feel the need to get charged and emotionally engaged, recite the words, sing the lines, or picture the face and message of the person you admire, and devote your efforts to your inspiration of choice.

Personally, I am inspired by a 97 year old man who recently published his first book. I am inspired by Van Morrison and his soulful voice and lyrics. I am inspired by all the champion athletes who continue to teach me what I need to know, such as the lessons of diligence, dedication, and devotion to a cause. I am inspired by nature's awesome gift of beauty as I mountain bike or run high in the Rockies on a balmy summer morning. Who or what inspires you, and how do you access this for future performance, work, practice, and life?

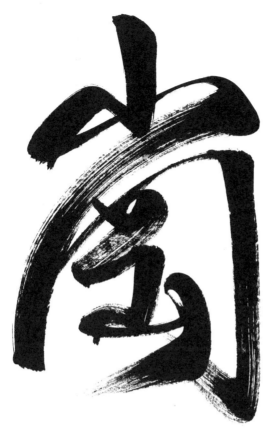

POSITION OF THE GRAY HERON

The following segment on the Great Gray Heron was given to me recently by my dear friend and administrative assistant, Sally Vaughn. Her sense of timing is impeccable. As I read the passage, I immediately thought, this is really about how we need to be as we attempt to coach with heart. Here it is:

> *The Great Gray Heron is all about Positioning. This magnificent creature is genetically wired to be poised, composed, and in perfect position, ready to strike when opportunity presents itself, ready for positive possibilities, and when challenges (pain, setbacks, loss) present themselves. We*

humans, on the other hand, often miss out on the opportunities for growth and positive change because, unlike the Heron, we focus on the distractions in our lives. We are often not ready or aware that change is needed, or that opportunity is knocking. Descriptions of the Heron include serene, easy, vigilant, lucid, contemplative, moving in the flow, unperturbed, and aware. All of these are ways of being, of living, of leading and coaching. These ways allow for openness. And it is that openness that permits us to embrace an opportunity and move forward in our lives, to help us reflect on and reevaluate situations as they present themselves. When the Heron is being this way, it captures its prey, gets what it needs.

Take ten minutes and reflect upon this passage. Answer the question: in what way is this paragraph on the Heron related to the purpose of the book you have in your hands? How are the ways of the Heron related to the ways of coaching with heart? What is the significance of the ways of the Heron to your coaching and overall life?

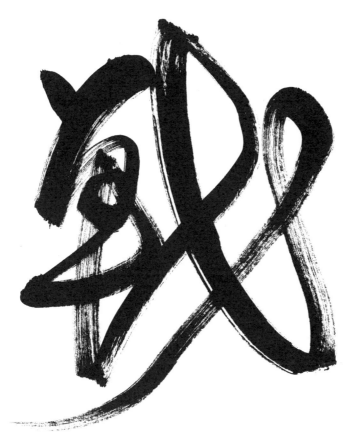

THE HEART OF WAR

Having been intimately involved in the arena of athletics as an athlete, coach, and sports psychologist for over 50 years, I now believe that there is one astounding truth that if taken to heart, will drastically alter your relationship with sports. It's not about winning, it's about competing for something bigger and more important than beating your opponent. When you and your team fight and battle for the love and respect of each other and refuse to sacrifice the gift that you've been given—health, strength, talent, friendship, family, and opportunity—you will be very difficult to beat. Heart-driven athletic cultures know that this is the only goal. To accomplish this, your athletes must commit to doing the best they can each day to be the very best they can be, so that they position themselves for their utmost best performance and possible victory. This is a daily commitment to excellence in practice and competition. Winning on the scoreboard is simply a reflection of achieving that daily goal.

Competing for something bigger than oneself means focusing on the process, not the outcomes; the controllable, not the uncontrollable; the love of the game and the team, not the fear of losing; giving, not taking; thinking outside-the-box, not traditionally. Competing for something bigger than simply a win means doing what others are not willing to do, to sacrifice and even suffer along the way. It is having one rule, and that is, to do the right thing even when others are not looking. When you compete, you're difficult to beat. Use this as a mantra, reminding you to focus on only that which you can control…all of the elements of competing.

As an exercise, help your team to compete with heart by doing the following: break the team up into small groups of five. (More or less, depending on the size of the team.) Ask each group to list five to ten specific ways that, when executed, demonstrate what it means to compete. For example, in basketball, you can dive for the ball, crash the boards, box out, sprint the lanes, and play "in your face" tenacious defense, all of which are controllable, doable, and easy to accomplish. When the groups have their answers, open the discussion to the entire team and create a master list that contains all of those competitive elements. Then, together, boil the entire list down to a roux, a collection of the thickest, richest, and most vital ways to compete. Allow this list to act as your team's competitive touchstone, a reference point to a culture that competes in this way.

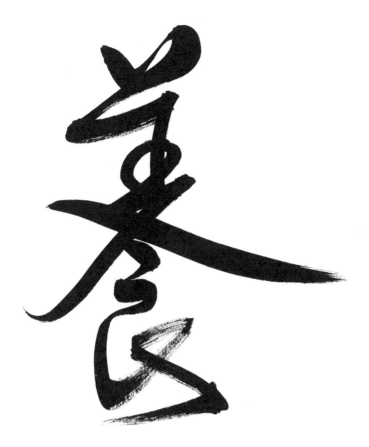

FERTILIZING THE SOIL

The wisdom of the Tao reminds us to care for all seeds ready to sprout, to encourage all shoots to reach for the sky, to offer nurturance and encouragement to flower and feed the hunger of the heart.

This process of nurturance I refer to is the fertilization of the "soil" of the heart, the feeding of the soul. When cultivating a young rose bush, we foster the new life in fertile soil, give it plenty of water and sunshine, and prune it appropriately, thereby encouraging rapid, healthy growth. From a simple seed comes a beautiful fragrant flower because we took the time and effort to nurture it throughout its growth process. This is no different from the process of coaching

with a dancing heart. Coaches, who affirm and nurture greatness within the athletes, create a place of hope and inspiration—a place where the soil is fertile for healthy growth and
change and high level performance.

The instinct to nurture is most obvious in parenting. All
parents can bring to the process this instinctual love and affection that they express toward children, especially during
moments of insecurity. In turn, they are greatly rewarded
when the same kind of caring and affection is reciprocated
from their children. It is an act of true giving and receiving,
serving one another "soul food."

With heart-directed coaching, nurturance implies the instilling of courage, giving athletes permission to follow their
heart, their passion, in all that they do amid the challenges
and tests in sport and life. Nurturance helps us to see how
nature conspires to provide what we need in our work; doors
seem to open to us that never opened before when we truly
follow the dancing heart of coaching.

The Chinese symbols for nurturance illustrate the process
of rainwater fertilizing the soil, making nature grow, and the
instinctual behaviors of all of us to nurture our young. It's a
foundational building block for effective coaching.

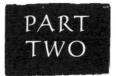

PART
TWO

WISDOM TO EMPOWER

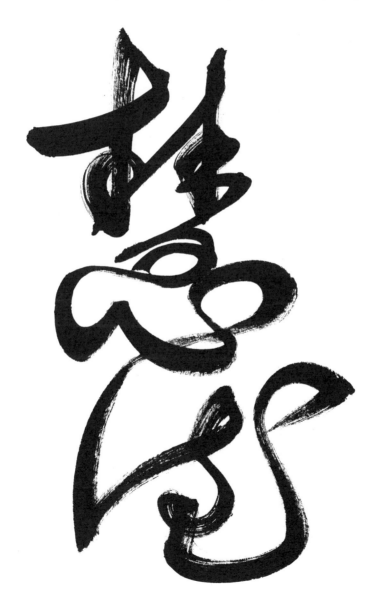

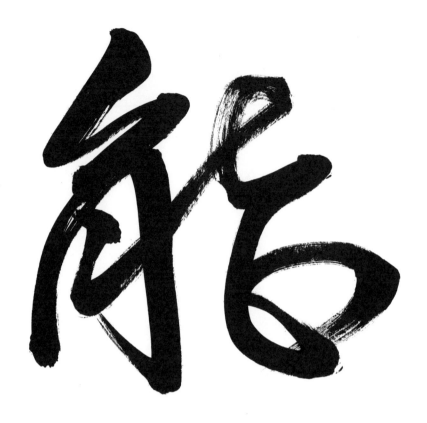

THREE NOBLE TALENTS

Let me remind you of the memorable over-time women's soccer World Cup competition between the USA and Japan. The story is not so much about Japan's victory as it was about why and how they won. Prior to the start of the OT period, the camera crew focused on both team huddles. The USA women's body language indicated to many of us deep concern, tightness of posture, perhaps indicating fear. I could be wrong, but they seemed to me to be overly concerned about fighting and battling for contracts with professional organizations. The Japanese, on the other hand, were smiling, laughing, seemingly confident and eager to fight and battle for the honor, privilege, and love of country, a higher more spiritually focused motivation, something much bigger than they themselves or the game itself. I knew at that moment that Japan would win. It's been my experience that coaches who inspire their athletes to compete for a deeper, more meaningful purpose and work much harder see them develop into a team that plays with heart, a team that demonstrates what I call, the *Three Noble Talents* of athletics.

First, there is *physical* talent. In the above contest, many would arguably say that the USA had more going for them on this level than Japan. At the very least, both teams were fairly well matched. Physical talent at this level probably accounts for about 10% of the outcome. It is important to have it yet the difference between these opponents physically was negligible.

The second of the three *Noble Talents* revolves around the *mental* game: who is mentally tougher and stronger? When the going gets tough, the tough get going. In today's athletic culture at this level, it is not uncommon for teams to employ personal sports psychologists to work on team building and develop solid mental training programs for high level performance. I have worked with over 120 national and international teams in this capacity for the last 25 years. Since so many athletic organizations are gaining this advantage, it can no longer be thought about as such. The mental piece probably accounts for another 30% of the outcome.

The remaining 60% of the outcome can be attributed to the third *Noble Talent*, the *spiritual* component. This is where the bulk of my work comes into play. I'm referring to the spirituality of performance, the courage, commitment, patience, persistence, perseverance, tenacity, integrity, cohesiveness, caring, love, connection, trust, respect, and sense of a higher more meaningful purpose to the battle, as we saw with the Japanese women and staff at the World Cup.

The *Three Noble Talents* are essential components to your sacred calling if you want to help your athletes discover their individual and collective greatness. In a recent contest between the same two countries at the 2012 Olympic games in London, the USA reversed the outcome against Japan in soccer as they seem to be more spiritually fit, fighting for a higher purpose of love and pride in country.

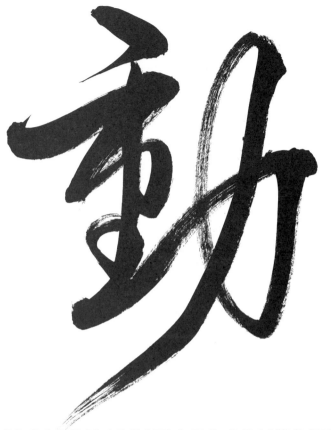

FROM DISABILITY TO POSSIBILITY

Sunryu Suzuki, in his classic bestseller, *Zen Mind, Beginner's Mind*, points out that "in the beginner's mind there are many possibilities; in the expert's mind, there are only a few." Experts are too "filled up" to see the options. Beginners, on the other hand, see nothing but joy, excitement, fun, and the multitude of alternatives. The beginner is a neophyte with a child's view, playing for the love of playing, like in a sandbox, free of judgment, pressure, and the fear of failure. It is a heart-based approach filled with passion and love. The more you enable your athletes to be in this emotional-spiritual space, the more you free them to play and compete up to their capacity, to focus on possibility rather than disability. Here are some ideas, strategies, and thoughts I have learned over the years that coaches use to help themselves coach with heart getting their athletes to compete in similar fashion as they open up to vast possibilities.

First of all, let me say that many of your athletes, over the years, have developed preconceived biases and beliefs that could seriously impede their performance. Many athletes back in the early 1950s believed that breaking the four-minute barrier in the mile run was impossible. Yet this limited belief was quickly shattered as champion Roger Bannister, keeping a beginner's open mind, did what the experts believed to be impossible.

To begin to help your athletes open their hearts and be nonjudgmental, ask them to write out a list of their favorite limiting beliefs, such as "I can't," "It never could happen," "I'm (we're) not good enough," and on and on. Help them to see the ways in which they act like experts, with no basis for proof. Now, using a beginner's mind, have them change these statements around (example: "I can...") and then list ways that demonstrate possibility rather than disability. A pertinent guiding question that will help them stay open to such possibility is: If you freed yourself to play up to your capacity, what do you think would be possible?

Another related approach I take in my coaching is to tell athletes that this could be their day for major breakthroughs. I ask them: "If you freed yourself to play up to capacity, what specifically needs to be done to make that come true?" Regardless of what happens, their nervous systems are aligned with openness and receptivity to possibility. They begin to seek out ways to fulfill the dream.

I like the concept of "new beginnings," which reinforces

the Zen mind approach. For example, in golf, if you hit a poor shot, approach the ball for the second shot and tell yourself that "here is a new beginning, a chance to start again and demonstrate how a champion, world-class golfer hits a ball." In tennis, each point becomes a new possibility, a new beginning. In soccer, each possession is a new start. Each half in lacrosse is a new game. Come out after halftime and play as if the score is zero-zero, whether you are up or down. After each mistake, error or failure, begin again. "New beginnings" becomes a theme throughout the entire match or game. Having this as a pre-game strategy is a relaxing way to begin the contest.

John Lilly, a psychologist researching dolphin behavior patterns, said that "beliefs are limits to be examined and transcended." When you observe dolphins in the wild, you can get a sense about what I mean by the beginner's mind. I am quite fortunate as I get to see these water athletes per-forming off shore a block from my home in California on an evening walk or run.

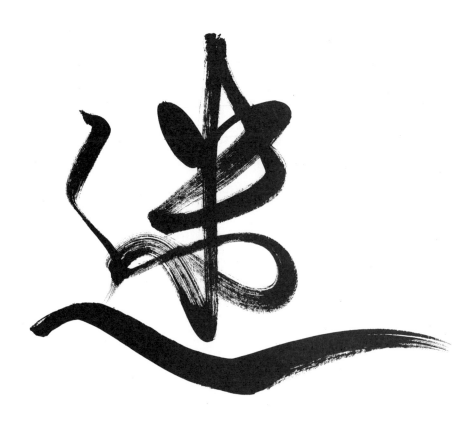

KEYS TO AUTHENTICITY

Over the lifespan of my professional career in various aspects of sports, I can confidently say that thousands of athletes have felt deep disappointment, dislike, and disrespect for their coaches. My take about one of the causes of these stress producing and performance debilitating feelings is the serious lack of authenticity on the part of the coach. What they seem to desire is a coach who is first and foremost, an authentic human being, not a "role." They crave (and I have been told this from the majority of these elite performers) a relationship with someone who cares (wouldn't you?). They want to be positively regarded, recognized, respected, relished, and valued for their contribution to the system. In order for a coach to cultivate authenticity in the relationship, there must be love in his or her heart. (See segment in Part I, Having Love in Your Heart.) As I mentioned before, no love, no coaching—it's that simple. The key is to give athletes the attention they need and deserve. This may require you to be more like a good, caring parent at times. Look your athletes in the eye, truly listen to them; touch them on the shoulder or pat them on the back. Be present with what is happening right now, as if they are the only important people in your life. Just be you and let your imagined role slip away. Work at letting your presence be simple, comfortable, natural, modest, humble, and unassuming. Other ways to cultivate authenticity are to acknowledge your weaknesses, shortcomings, and past failures. Also, give credit to others when credit is due, especially when you hadn't thought about their good ideas. Become comfortable with speaking truths, especially when they are not popular. Let others know that you relish and invite feedback. Many coaches fear or refuse to hear such critiques.

I notice how so many who call themselves coaches act superior, play a role, and fear that if they be themselves, they will not be good enough or that somehow, they will lose control. So they hide, pose, pretend, posture, and play the part and, in the process, lose authenticity and become unconscious in a "game without purpose." They fill their egos while emptying their souls. They sacrifice their potential positive influence. Echkart Tolle, in his insightful book, *A New Earth*, points out that a role is the ego creating separation. Emotional engagement, so essential for coaching with a dancing heart, is impossible when you separate yourself by playing a role. People play roles because they may feel insecure. It is like wearing a mask; some feel they can't work without one, but in actuality one can't do the important work with it.

What I have learned over the years is that when I put my role aside and am myself, being vulnerable, present, transparent, and authentic, I have a subtle transformational effect on whomever I coach and lead. I am most powerful (not power over others), most influential, most effective, and most happy when I am being completely myself. And the nice thing about that is: I am not superior to anyone, nor inferior. I refuse to take myself too seriously.

What I notice about so many who "play the role" of leader-coach is that they do take themselves and life much too seriously. When this occurs, the spontaneity, joy, lightheartedness and humor become invisible (assuming these traits ever existed). In the absence of such authenticity, true, effective, inspirational leadership is not possible. Humorless, joyless leadership is an oxymoron. Basically, the "role" itself begins to define you as a "human doing"; you lose touch with the real you, a "human being" having a leadership experience, not a leader having a human experience. You may have noticed how many doctors, because of total identification with their role, can only relate to others as case loads, or "the heart case in room 117." Such impersonalization leads to doctor/patient interactions that are unauthentic and at times, outright dehumanizing. If you lose yourself in the "role of leader-coach," you run the risk of not having authentic relationships with those whom you guide. Remember that extraordinary leadership/coaching is all about the creation of safe, trustworthy, respectful, human being relationships. Authentic, emotionally engaging relationships are impossible to create when you get too self-absorbed and lost in the role. Be a human being who is working in a leadership capacity and really understand that when you buy into "the role model," you prevent yourself from being an inspiration-al, empowering, and influential leader. The way to ensure authenticity is through awareness. Be aware of how you talk and interact and treat those you guide, if you desire to be influential. Is your role and the subsequent way you relate to others causing distance, making you feel superior, prevent-ing emotional engagement? Is it a block to being transparent when transparency actually facilitates the power of authen-ticity, the way of influence in all relationships for effective guidance? My wife, Jan, is an amazing person and a doctor—she doesn't wear a white coat (fly her "Role Flag," as it were).

When students are confused about how to address me, I tell them, "if it doesn't interfere with your education, call me Jerry—that's who I am." I gain their respect, trust, and their following because of who I really am, not my socially sanc-tioned title of "Doctor." I must let go of self definitions and focus on being what I really am, a human being coaching others to be something other than ordinary.

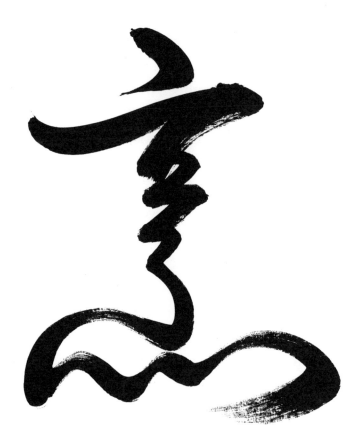

LIKE FRYING A DELICATE FISH

So many times during my coaching career or days as a Naval officer, I have operated or led from a place of fear—the fear of losing control over those I lead. This need I had to control came from what I believe was a basic sense of personal insecurity, of believing that to be successful, I must force, manipulate, or coerce others into doing it my way. Farmers have learned through experience that if you want to control the cows, move the fences back. Only when I was willing to let go of excessive control did I, my team, and others enjoy true learning and victory. Confucius says that great leaders "guide others and do not pull them along; urge them to go forward by opening the way, yet refuse to take them there."

The *Tao* teaches, as I have stated earlier in the book, that true leadership is to lead like you fry a delicate fish—lightly. Restriction, rules, and regulations should be used but sparingly. Too many controls are not only difficult to enforce, they create counter-reactions from those being controlled and paradoxically, the leader loses control. "Make smart boundaries, be firm within those, and give others the chance to breathe and let their creative juices flow." This quote taken from the *Tao Te Ching* reminds us that it's all about those you lead, not you, the leader. You are certainly aware of coaches who micro-manage incessantly and fail to see the big picture of developing, orchestrating, and choreographing a highly productive, creative, and functional environment. *Control* stifles the process of extraordinary leadership because those they lead will find ways to sabotage all of your efforts to gain control. They will feel anger and resentment and lose respect for you. *Control* is a form of manipulation that creates distrust and suspicion. Motivation and team spirit diminish in controlling environments. It's much better to set wise limits and then turn them loose as they discover their own greatness. As a leader and coach you need your students and athletes as much as they need you. And remember the Golden Rule: treat others as you would like to be treated. Create the delicate balance between all-out control and none at all.

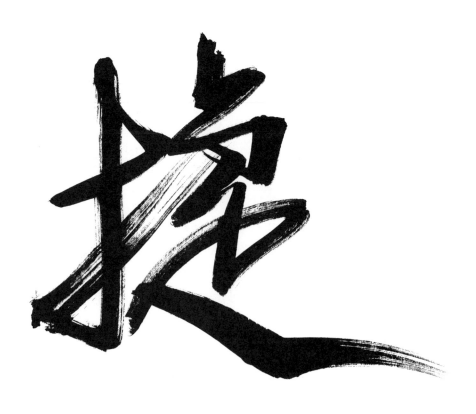

FAST FOOD OR SOUL FOOD

Most leaders who have control issues are using what seems to be an industrial model, a linear, authoritative approach based on conformity. They seem to "manufacture" good soldiers who follow orders. The heart leader, on the other hand, uses a creative agricultural model, one that is organic in nature not mechanical. They are able to establish environments where others will flourish. They are willing and able to "customize" conditions to the circumstances of a situation depending on individual differences and needs. With such personalized leadership, they "grow" protégés who, rather than follow orders like a good soldier, follow their hearts. The difference between the two styles is drastic: the first model is akin to eating greasy "fast food" while that of the heart leader feeds on organic, healthy gourmet fare. The former is more physically and spiritually costly. The latter energizes, inspires, and empowers the spirit with good "soul food." What model do you prefer? Can I take your order?

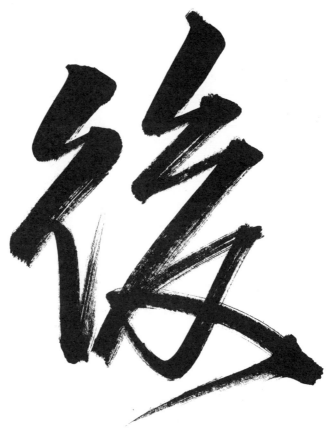

PUTTING YOURSELF LAST

Evolved Individuals put themselves last,
and yet they are first.
Put themselves outside, and yet they remain.
Is it not because they are without self-interest
That their interests succeed?

Tao Te Ching no. 7

In an ancient Eastern story, heaven and hell are exactly alike: Each is an enormous banquet where the most incredible, delectable dishes are placed on huge tables. Those who partake in the feast are given chopsticks *five feet long*. In the banquet in hell, people give up struggling to feed themselves with these awkward utensils and remain ravenously unfulfilled. In heaven, everyone selflessly feeds the person across the table.

According to the *Tao*, those who are in the background will eventually be brought forward. Even in the Judeo-Christian tradition, the meek—the truly humble, unboastful, selfless people—will be recognized as worthy. Lao-Tzu encourages action without self-interest; selflessness ultimately brings personal fulfillment. As a coach, the most important question you can ask is: How can I give to my athletes, my team, and staff?

Selflessness is an active process of devotion to others' welfare and interests—even sometimes at the expense of your own. Giving to your team enhances your own coaching performance as they look for ways to reciprocate. Bring out another's best, give praise, and the same will be provided for you over and over. What you give, you get back.

A professional athlete who epitomizes selflessness is basketball great Tim Duncan of the San Antonio Spurs. I have seen him pass the ball to a trailing player during a fast break when he could have easily taken the layup himself. He takes a sincere interest in helping the younger players on the team improve. Because of this, players throughout the NBA have the utmost respect for him. He gives so much, yet he gets back a hundredfold from the admiration of his peers and certainly his fans.

Selflessness is personal power. Taoists call it *tz'u*, which means "caring." It is caring for others' performances, individually and as a team. The more you give to your athletes, the more you possess. Teams with a selfish coach experience much friction and anxiety that detract from team unity and performance, but selflessness creates peace and conserves energy, which allows for higher levels of play from your athletes.

The more you can model an environment of selflessness, the greater the chances of your athletes becoming like you. This, ultimately, impacts how your team performs. High performing teams are selfless teams. Bill Bradley, basketball star with Princeton University and the New York Knicks, knows about the impact of selflessness on a team's performance. In his beautiful book, *Values of The Game*, Bradley claims that "championships are not won unless a team has forged a high degree of unity, attainable only through the selflessness of each of its players. Untrammeled individualism destroys the chance for achieving victory."

Strange but true, when the name on the front of the jersey is more important than the name on the back, amazing things happen. When a team shifts from a "me" focus to a "we" consciousness, they achieve at higher levels. I'm not sure where I heard this, but I use it often: T.E.A.M. is an acronym for "together everyone achieves more."

Being selfless is similar to a good investment. Invest in your team, and as the "heart" account grows, and you refuse to withdraw from it, you accumulate dividends payable down the road. The rewards are certain, you just need to trust.

And trusting this is not easy for any of us. At times it seems counterintuitive. It's natural for your athletes to fear that they won't get what they deserve. But in time, you as their coach will begin to see that this higher road of selflessness and giving is the one you will always want to take. You will never master the art of selflessness and giving. Just try to be more conscious of it and give more often.

When you find yourself hesitating to give, for whatever reason, think about this story: The most selfless act one can perform is to risk one's own life trying to save the life of another. When San Antonio Spurs star Sean Elliot was in dire need of a kidney transplant, his brother Noel selflessly stepped up and saved Sean's life.

In his book *Man's Search for Meaning*, Viktor Frankl gives us a vivid dramatic example of the spiritual sustenance provided by being selfless. While incarcerated in a Nazi death camp, Frankl noted that the people who kept their strength and sanity the longest were not the ones who managed by force or cleverness to obtain more than their share of scarce food. Instead it was those who aided other prisoners and shared selflessly with them the little food they had. Their physical and mental condition seemed to be strengthened by their selflessness, by the focus placed on their fellow prisoners rather than themselves. The outcome is no different when athletes adopt this virtue as a way of being with a team.

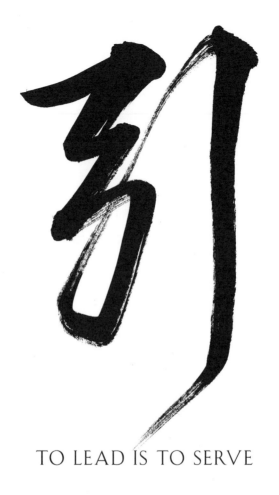

TO LEAD IS TO SERVE

Paraphrasing an ancient Chinese proverb: to lead is to serve, to serve is to lead. Perhaps the strongest objective of the dancing heart coach is service, surrendering oneself for the greater good of others. Service is the focal point and sacred purpose of effective guidance. What I have observed from my years in leadership roles coupled with watching, listening to, and working with extraordinary leaders and coaches is that service requires both a give and take from all involved in the relationship; athletes give to their coaches what coaches need to know, so that, in turn, coaches can give back to the athletes what they need in order to accomplish a task. This is one important part of the dance I refer to in a previous section, Wu Shi Leadership.

In Japanese, the word samurai means "service with heart, honor, and integrity." In this sense, the ideal coach or leader is akin to the samurai, one who serves, guides, and leads with heart. Service as such is not about servitude or catering to all wishes of those you lead. It is about valuing those you lead and adding worth to their lives. As a coach, you are in charge and oversee the big picture but you offer your service by providing an honorable environment with integrity for all to reach their potential. Such service-oriented coaches refuse to micro-manage and exert control as this leads to mistrust, lack of cooperation, loss of faith, diminished enthusiasm, and the unwillingness of others to "go the distance." Once again, Chief Oren Lyons, in an interview called "Leadership Imperative" says that the purpose of leadership is to serve others. It appears that the most effective leaders examine their hearts and ask the question: am I here to serve or to be served? Obviously it's to serve. Therefore, the most important question that a heart-directed leader and coach needs to ask is "how can I best serve you?" When you follow the answer to this simple query, those you lead will experience a heightened sense of self and you, as a result, gain more power, not over people, but the power to influence and dance with them, and help facilitate change and growth for all involved. This is why we say, "to serve is to lead."

Serving others, you must remember, requires that you trust and treat them with respect, compassion and love, thus enhancing the chances of positive results. The *I Ching* tells us:

"Service towards others will create a spirit of unparalleled loyalty. Followers will take on much hardship and suffering toward the attainment of goals."

Fundamentally, such service and heart-directed work places the well-being of humanity above the well-being of those who lead. The well-known Russian novelist Leo Tolstoy once said: "The sole purpose of life is to serve humanity. It is the honorable and right thing to do." And, in the process of this service, you become more respected, loved, and worthy as you enhance the lives of all those whom you lead.

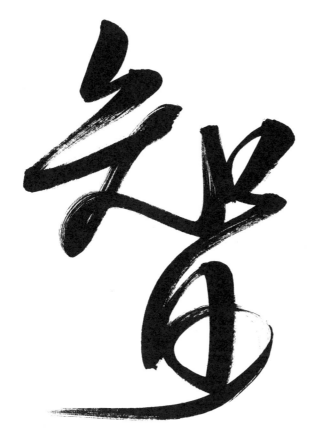

CONSCIOUS SELF AWARENESS

The strength of a heart-directed coach is the propensity for self-knowledge, an "insightful strength" that provides an accurate appraisal of who you are as well as your levels of mental, emotional, and spiritual fitness. It's important to know your game and know your athletes and when this knowledge is combined with an inner knowing, your best work will be possible. Chinese sage Sun-Tzu, in *The Art of War*, talks about such inner awareness. To paraphrase his thoughts, when you know both yourself and your athletes, you are in the best place to lead and coach. Know the athletes but not yourself and you have half a chance of being effective. Knowing neither puts you in a bad position.

You will be most effective as a coach when you are aware of your strengths and weaknesses as well as those of your athletes. I suggest that periodically, have the courage to take an accurate inventory of your personal struggles, the obstacles that stand in your way, recurrent fears and frustrations, and determine where the most work is needed in order to go beyond these self-imposed limitations. Knowing yourself is a way to develop confidence and poise. It is a hedge against selling yourself short as a leader and to feel personally proud of who you are, where you've been, and where you are going in your professional life. Know, for instance, that you have within you right now, all that you need to be the very best coach possible. You deserve to be the best you can be. And, remember, this is all very true for those athletes whom you love and coach. Knowing yourself helps you to help them in this way.

Involved in the process of personal development is the concept of self-acceptance where you must create positive self-images and self-talk, pictures and words that clearly spell out your strengths while creating a vision of what is possible. Replace old, worn-out negative thoughts and messages with up-beat positive phrases and affirmations that are forward moving and facilitate your upward development as a heart-directed coach. This becomes an ongoing updating process to avoid listening to the deleterious chatter of negativity. Following the advice of the I Ching, "you should exercise unrelenting discipline over your thought patterns. Cultivate only productive attitudes."

Let me suggest three poignant soul-searching questions to get you started on your quest of conscious self-knowing and awareness (as a coach, as a person).

1. What do you like about yourself? Please blow your own horn a bit.
2. What do you dislike about yourself? Please be brutally honest.
3. What can you do to change any item in #2 so that it gets listed in #1?

Have some fun with this exercise. Write the positive affirmations on index cards and recite them every day. Trust me, this works.

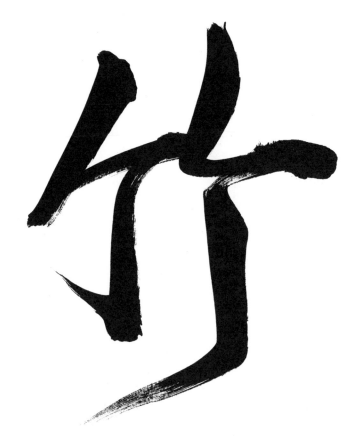

THE BAMBOO WAY

Those who are firm and inflexible
are in harmony with dying.
Those who are yielding and flexible
are aligned with living.

Tao Te Ching no. 76

Bamboo is elegant, strong, and versatile and flourishes in all hostile conditions: rain, wind, snow, or even in constant foot traffic when used as a beautiful kitchen floor. Its flexible nature helps it to adapt to change, perform at higher levels, and avoid extinction.

Like bamboo, the physically, mentally, emotionally, spiritually strong and flexible dancing heart coach will endure and realize full growth and development as well as triumph along the path to realizing personal greatness.

Let's begin on the physical plane. To be a model for growth and change, it is crucial to consistently stretch one's muscles and connective tissue. Loose, fluid bodies are less prone to injury and illness. This is particularly essential to maintaining vibrancy as we age. A coach who is less than vibrant is less effective with those under his or her tutelage. A strong, healthy, and flexible body is the perfect home for your spirit and soul. Modeling this sends a good message to others who work with you to better themselves. Good modeling is good coaching.

As coaches who serve with a dancing heart, we want to guard against inflexibility of the mind. Rigid beliefs about what we and our followers can or cannot do are self-imposed limits that need to be examined and transcended. Failure to do so will align you with loss, mistakes, failure, and fear. For example, when you and those you coach use the inflexible reactive words "I can't" you sabotage any willingness to do all that is possible to go beyond your limited belief. Changing these words to "I can do it, I am strong" is a powerful, flexible proactive affirmation that gives you permission to test your body's capability to actually go beyond what you once thought were limits.

Also, being inflexible stands in the way of adapting to sudden, unexpected change. In all of life, change is the only constant. Your failure to adapt to inevitable change prevents you from performing to your capacity as well as holding back those whom you serve and coach. Your greatest quality as a heart-directed coach in all arenas is a quiet adaptation to change, be it during a competitive event, a family matter, a business transaction, or some other mercurial situation.

Be pliable, fluid, and bending like bamboo. Examine what

have been your rigid beliefs and challenge them on all fronts. Create a fluidity of body, mind, and spirit. Notice the difference in your work performance as well as those with whom you work, when you are more relaxed, flexible, and fluid versus when you are fearful, tight, and tense during times of inevitable change.

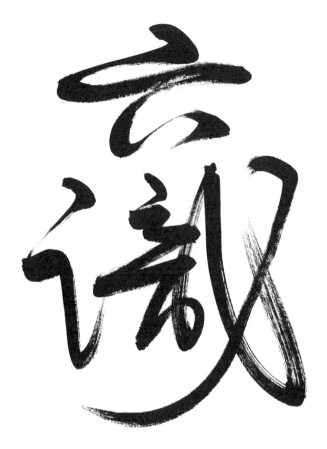

SIXTH SENSE OF SACRED AWARENESS

It is knowing without knowing. It is a subconscious gut feeling. Some think of it as a mystical power. Others talk about it as instinct or an opening to your sixth sense. But scientists who study this phenomenon refer to it as the inner powers of the mind. In a word: *Intuition*. In the *Tao Te Ching*, Lao-Tzu writes about intuition being the purest form of information. According to *Webster's New World Dictionary*, intuition is defined as "the direct knowing or learning of something without the conscious use of reasoning." It is real knowledge and immediate knowing based on wisdom accrued from your extraordinary coaching and life experiences. This "gut feeling," your inner voice, comes from many hours of studying, strategizing, and planning how to respond to real life situations. Dancing heart coaches are in tune with intuitive leadership.

The *I Ching* reminds us to "act out the dance of your inner self, trust the inherent correctness of your instincts…in this way you will meet with success." Over the years, I have learned that to know and to act are one and the same. Your actions and performance are the result of the body's innate intelligence, coupled with a mind that trusts what the body knows while being willing to step out of the way. It is a response that comes from our unconscious minds. Martial artists call this sixth sense a state of hyperawareness that produces calm in an otherwise fearful, tense situation. In sports, fitness, and life, performance is directly related to your ability to follow your inner intuitive sense, those impulses, feelings, and automatic responses—quick reactions in fast-paced situations.

All great coaches and athletes trust their intuition. Whether making split-second decisions, anticipating a fastball, knowing what to do or when to surge in a race, positioning yourself to catch a pass, or reacting to a defense or an offense, while coaching a big game you need to call upon and trust your intuitive self. Meditation practice (see segment *Strength of Ten Tigers*) will help you to develop and strengthen your intuition.

We all possess this instinct, yet few of us trust it to the extent we must to be consistently successful. When we are in the midst of leading and coaching others, there is often no time to think; you need to cultivate and develop your instincts as you coach, lead, practice, and work out. Follow your inner voice and notice how things develop. Know that good things happen when you rely on natural insight.

Instinct, or intuitive action, is a significant aspect of Zen and Buddhist thinking, and an integral part of coaching with heart. Notice how your greatest successes occur during those times when you trust the wisdom of your heart, your basic instinct. Paraphrasing the words of the *Tao Te Ching*, evolved individuals know without going about, recognize without looking, achieve without acting, and follow their hearts.

Missy Foote, head women's lacrosse coach at Middlebury College faced a dilemma after a significant loss prior to her team entering the conference tournament championship. Her assistants and others had her questioning the plan, the system, and approach they had used to be so successful all season, just out of fear following that defeat. She and I had talked about this and when we were finished, she concluded that she had the feeling that it was best to follow her instincts, to trust the athletes and what had worked all season. She did that and Middlebury went on to win the conference title and got to eventually play in the NCAA Championship game for the 15th time.

Those coaches who have a "feel" for making the right decision at the right time are more than lucky. They have developed over time a special understanding of their sport and the many factors specific to the circumstances at hand. How can you creatively develop this intuitiveness in your own program? Begin to trust yourself and your experiences in your sport and in working with your athletes.

You can be much more effective when you act according to the laws of your inner self and trust the inherent correctness of your intuition when solving problems, making decisions, and answering questions. Ask yourself *What feels right?* Give the answer some weight. You can combine this with input from others or take more time to analyze the situation. Many of us needlessly search for solutions to problems by going "outside" ourselves and following ways that simply do not feel right. Perhaps you've been coaching your sport for a number of years, and before that you were an athlete. You really do know how to act in most situations; you need to trust and follow that inner voice and see for yourself that you knew all along what was the right thing to do. It takes courage and practice, but the payoffs will reward you.

When you stop second-guessing yourself, you become more confident, consistent, and happier with your work and relationships with your athletes. Doing what feels right is as important as doing what you rationally know may be right. We need to take both aspects—intuitive feelings and rational thought—into account when making our decisions. If our intuitive sense seems stronger, give more attention to it. Being adaptable to situations and open to change is also part of intuitiveness. When you get the chance to intuitively act on something in coaching, take the risk and follow your innate wisdom and notice the outcome. This behavior requires practice; in time you'll discover its value.

You may already realize that there has been a strong movement in corporate circles to rely on the heart in the decision-making process behind multimillion-dollar business deals. Intuitive management is encouraged by CEOs who understand the value of inner wisdom as a guiding force. The same inner wisdom is valuable for coaches as well. And, even if you are a relatively new coach, you possess such inner wisdom. You are probably a warehouse of athletic knowledge; just remember that and trust your wisdom. Use it often and pair it with a look at the data and the results. Train yourself through experimentation to become more confident and less fearful. Start out with smaller decisions and go with what you feel to be right. Gradually work up to those you believe are the bigger decisions and notice the confidence you feel.

The next time you're confronted with a difficult decision, a problem to solve or a question to answer, give your "inner mate" the bandwidth to solve the issue.

The Chinese symbols for instinct describe a direct entry into the very center of consciousness, with all instinctual senses open and focused to awaken the wisdom of inner knowing, what your heart knows to be right. Once again, Lao-Tzu wonders: "Can you give the wisdom of your heart precedence over the learning of your head?" The dancing heart coach does.

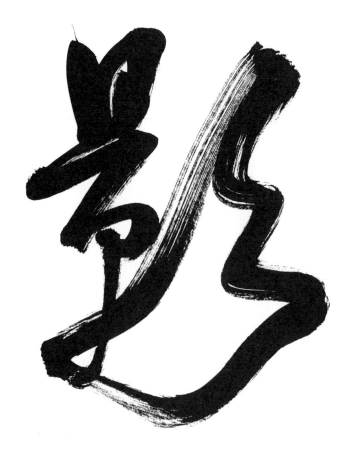

POWER OF INFLUENCE

I possess tremendous power to make life miserable or joyous. I can humiliate, humor, hurt, or heal. I am the decisive element. It is my personal approach that creates the climate.

Johann Wolfgang von Goethe

Perhaps the most challenging task of any coach is how to influence those they lead in a positive, forward moving manner. It is simple yet not easy; your influence can create or it can destroy; it can light a fire in an athlete's belly or it can douse the flames. Understand this: your influence is powerful yet never neutral. I am always aware of this when I compete, speak, teach, mentor, parent, or coach. My body language, my tone, my expressions, my gestures, my words all have an impact on how things transpire. As a coach, the more often you become aware of the power of your influ-

ence, the more you have a say in the outcome, the direction athletes will go, what they do, and how they feel. It is that simple. When I am coaching one of my teams I usually begin the sessions by inviting the athletes to "huddle up" close, forming a tight series of concentric circles (assuming there are 25 or so athletes on the team) around me. This communicates togetherness, kindness, oneness, connectedness, and, most importantly, a sense of goodness. There is no greater impact on your influence than goodness. It inspires and empowers others to move forward. I then proceed to mention how fortunate I am to be part of their lives and how happy I am being with them. I maintain good eye contact as I speak in a caring, warm tone. I may even touch a shoulder of an athlete to communicate caring if the moment presents itself. Being aware of this power to influence others is to coach with heart. The athletes love it; they respond in like manner. As I have learned, goodness inspires others and strengthens your positive influence. We then go back to where we were, sitting, standing, milling around and I have their full, undivided, respectful attention. By doing this, I set a positive, heart-directed tone for all the good work we will then do together.

When working with individual athletes, I love to maintain a powerful positive influence with (not over) them. To do so, I call on L.U.V.

L is for listen. I let them talk and listen intently to their issues or concerns. I notice how athletes respect coaches who listen to them. Listening, it turns out, is one of the more important keys to heart-based leadership. (Remember our discussion in *The Art of Listening?*)

U is to understand through the process of asking questions. I proceed to ask basic, direct questions based on what I've heard, helping them to gain clarity through their answers as well as enabling them to feel valued by my close connection to their important words.

Finally, V is for validate. Everyone wants to feel special and important and the validation process helps in this regard. Validation gives definition to the coaching environment, helping to inspire and empower the athlete to commit, persevere, compete, and comply with the team culture. It reinforces any and all success experiences, helping an athlete to stay on track and connected. I may say something like: "I appreciate your open candid remarks about the team. We value your input. You're important to our success." Or "I am so happy you brought that to my attention. I'm glad you are part of this team." Know that these vital three entities, L.U.V. are interdependent and dance together with no particular order.

Another way that I expand the power of my influence is by focusing on being confident in my knowledge, skill-set, wisdom, and experience in a kind and generous giving way. Being comfortable in my own skin, something that took years for me to achieve, strengthens my confidence. People are attracted to those who are confident. When I feel confident, I have a more positive influence to generate among my athletes and coaches.

As you can see, the power of your influence is something to be aware of at all times. Your influence is directly related to the relationships developed by you with your athletes. The next segment will go into more detail about this thought.

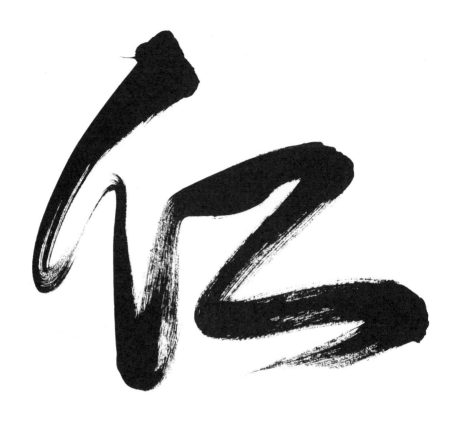

WINNING THE RELATIONSHIP GAME

Extraordinary heart-directed coaching begins and ends with one word: Relationships, the single most vital aspect to successful coaching. Top coaches have figured out that the way to get ahead is not necessarily to win games but to win the relationship game. These relationships are cultivated in emotionally safe environments where deep caring, love, respect, and integrity are forged, where failure is a learning opportunity and athletes are not fearful of taking risks, making mistakes, and losing. Such "sacred spaces" teach that we may lose, but by so doing, we really win. In these environments, the communication of caring, dancing heart coaches becomes the bridge to building strong, healthy relationships. They know that when you communicate well, you are truly invested in your athletes' success, and they have a much greater chance of reaching their full potential. When you communicate your belief in them, they are more inclined to "go the distance," to do all that you ask, to take appropriate risks and to get going when the going gets tough. As I have stated earlier in the book, athletes don't care about what you know, they just want to know that you care. Such caring is built and solidified through communication, which in turn becomes the foundation for strong, positive relationships.

With a strong, positive relationship, you can ask your athletes to do all it takes to improve and they will oblige accordingly, provided you let them know that you have confidence in their ability to do it. They need to know, also, that if they fail, you will be there to help them to learn from the setback and coach them to eventually master it. I tell my athletes that I am here for them and will always have their best interest in mind.

It must be pointed out, however, that there is an important, fundamental first step in the establishment of solid relationships that cannot be overlooked. It is Trust. Do you remember the L.U.V. strategy in the Power of Influence? Good! When you develop this influence with your athletes, they will begin to trust their fearless leader. Here's how it works: when an athlete feels heard, understood, and validated, the athlete feels safer. When feeling safer, there is a feeling of trust. With more trust comes more openness. When an athlete is more open, learning increases and performance improves. The more an athlete opens to you the more influence you have and the more effective you will be with all those whom you lead. Simply put: No Trust, No Relation-ship. And I will let you in on a secret: trust is an essential aspect to extraordinary coaching; love is as well. Go back to Part I and re-read the section on *Having Love in Your Heart*.

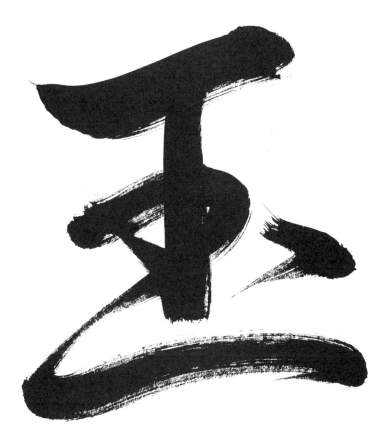

CONCEAL THE JADE

Do not boast overtly.
Keep the jade and treasures
reserved within the bosom.
A posture of humble heart will
bring blessings from all directions.

Tao Te Ching no. 24

Confucius tells the story of a warrior's display of humili-ty: when his people were defeated in battle, he was last to flee. People thought he was brave. So as to not look too boastful, he simply said that his staying behind was due only to the slowness of his horse; as a result, honor and glory were his. We are more appreciated when we are humble and choose to focus on others' greatness. The Tao virtue of Humility helps to ward off the need to claim credit or to be responsible for full success.

A beautiful example of such humility was John Wooden, coach of the UCLA Bruins. He often said that when his team wins, it is their doing; when they lose, it is his responsibility.

This is not to say that you cannot be proud of you or your team's achievements. Cherish the moment of recognition or victory. Celebrate your efforts while remaining aware that bragging and self-aggrandizement are the patterns of insecure coaches who need to promote themselves, yet find it difficult to live up to this inflated image.

To secure honor and glory, give recognition to the greatness of those around you. Notice how others on your team, on your staff, or at home, as well as your opponents, will return the gesture. Learning lessons of humility will help you to become a better coach and person in every aspect of life. There's no need for you to do anything to make others become aware of your greatness. That will happen by itself. When you really think about it, people are usually uncomfortable around those who brag or boast. Have you ever noticed how your unsolicited divulgence of your accomplishments, achievements, or advantages tends to be somewhat offensive, turning others against you? On the other hand, if others seem curious, you shouldn't hesitate to answer their questions and give them information about yourself that could further the conversation. Look for opportunities where you can sincerely affirm yourself and others.

Taoist thought encourages us to be all that we have been given, yet act as if we have nothing. In this way, no one will be aware of us yet we will bring happiness to all.

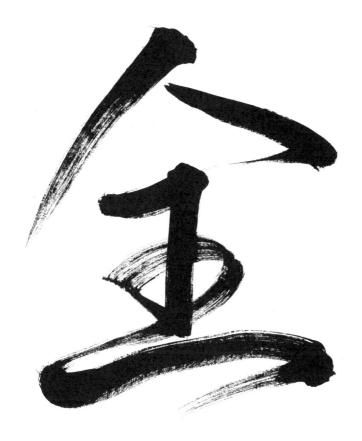

WHOLENESS OF CHARACTER

Hold to your ethics and principles.
Stand strongly for what you hold true.
Believe in your true self without compromises.
Trust in the power within yourself and use it.
Act in concert with your dreams and visions.

Tao Te Ching

To hold to your ethics and principles is to act with integrity. I define integrity as the narrowing of the gap between what we believe and say and what we do. It is, ultimately, doing the right thing. It is strength of character.

What happens when we trust our sense about what's

right, hold to our ethics and principles, and proceed to act on them in an honest fashion? Tao sages tell us that when we are true and honest to ourselves we hit upon what is right, find what is good, understand what's to be known, and create a life of harmony, happiness, satisfaction, and success.

Only by being true and honest to our inner selves can we fulfill our coaching dreams and those of our athletes. When we are out of touch with our inner self, we feel fear. So we must maintain our integrity at all costs by identifying and cultivating our deep-rooted values. Only by knowing what they are can we act with integrity. We allow others to control our thoughts or beliefs and make us feel inferior when we act dishonestly about these values. What would it be like if we acted from a place of deep self-truth to connect with the same deep truth with our teams? If being deeply honest threatens this relationship, do you really have a healthy thing going?

Integrity is the refusal to "sell out" on the true inner self, regardless of what situations in life present themselves; it is one of the most important aspects of coaching with heart.

When you gaze at the Chinese characters for the word integrity, it puts this virtue in perspective. Translated, they mean: "wholeness and refinement of character, denoting the commitment to stand up for personal principles, to keep oneself away from tainted influences and temptations."

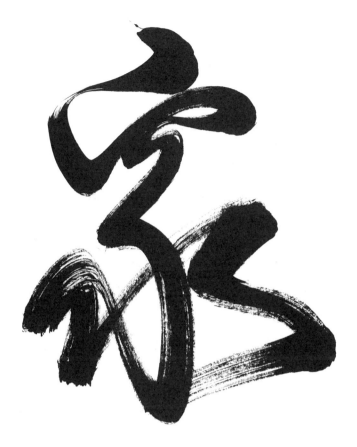

CULTURE OF WE NOT ME

Thus far, I have been engaged with you in the process of coaching with heart. Let's take some extended time to discuss and think about cultures of teams that are led with heart and how you, as their coach, can facilitate the development of such strong cultures, what they do, who they are, and how they behave and compete.

First of all, such heart-directed cultures are very much like a flock of geese migrating to warmer climates. These geese fly together, in a V formation, in selfless fashion to help each other to fly with less effort. When this happens, they can fly over seventy percent further than without working together. Your athletes need to hear about these birds.

Notice how these majestic aviators are continually communicating with each other the sweet sounds of encouragement and positive chatter; they could be saying "way to go, big bird, keep it up, looking strong, you can do it." Heart teams mimic their fine feathered friends in this way.

And perhaps most importantly, their communal, family-like behavior reflects the deep caring and compassion these creatures display for each other. When one of the family experiences injury or sickness during the journey, a small group of them stay behind to nurture their buddy back to health. They are present for each other during a crisis. So it is with heart-coached teams in a culture of selfless love and caring as they relieve each other's pain and help those in need.

When coaches model these behaviors for their teams, they perform at higher levels together. The wisdom of *The Art of War* tells us that a cohesive, unified team, well connected and competing with one heart and soul often will defeat a more talented group that lacks such qualities. From my experience with over 45 Final Four teams in various sports, there's nothing more satisfying and astounding than experiencing such a team of inspired, cohesive, well-cared for athletes playing together.

Strategist Sun-Tzu believed that the key to triumph in battle is unity of purpose and heart. In *The Art of War*, he states:

> Those who establish a viable group will win even if they are small. The key to all operations is harmony and connection with people.

Tao wisdom teaches that a culture of connection, team

spirit, and cohesion are vital aspects for victory both on the field and in all of life. In an age when many seem self-absorbed, when "me not we" is a mantra, we can use such wisdom and practice the virtue of selflessness in many ways.

Think of the cohesion demonstrated by the 1980 U.S. Olympic hockey team or the 1999 women's World Cup champion soccer team, whose hearts and souls were forged together on their journey to victory. Both teams were united by their willingness to embrace unity, oneness, and team spirit, placing these warriors in position to realize their dreams. I can honestly say that every one of the 29 national championship teams that I have had the honor and fortune to work with possess the quality of oneness, unified for a common goal of being a cohesive family. Creating team unity and cohesion for any coach takes work. Even if your team doesn't seem to possess natural team chemistry, this quality can be learned and instilled as a result of your heart-directed leadership as you model the exact behaviors for them to emulate.

Strong team cultures are well aware of how synergy and cooperative action impact success. It is the key to team effectiveness in any arena of life. In his insightful book *Playing for Keeps*, David Halberstam talks about how, at the University of North Carolina, under the guidance of coach Dean Smith, "everything was built around the concept of team… In the long run he believed that you went further by working as a team and sacrificing individuality to team effort…it would serve his players better later in their lives." Who could argue with such a successful program—and the success of its graduates twenty years later?

Furthering these thoughts, coach Phil Jackson believes

that good teams become great ones when they adopt the notion of selflessness, trust each other, and get beyond the "me" for the "we." He believes that the critical ingredient for a championship is love, the element of sharing, giving, and deep caring.

Students of history can point out how world cultures strive for spiritual togetherness, to harmonize the hearts and minds of the people. The *Tao Te Ching* reminds us that cultures that eternally exist do so because they exist for each other. Sports teams, business organizations, and families that exist for each other tend to be around for a long time.

The following strategies, tools, observations, and suggestions are taken from my vast experience over the past 30 years working with national championship cultures who compete with heart. Perhaps some of this will help you in your work with your athletes:

- Strong heart-felt cultures do not focus on winning championships and outcomes. Instead they focus on the mental process of building a strong foundation/culture that will ultimately create peak performance on a consistent basis, thus placing them in position to be the best they can be and, as a byproduct, win themselves a conference, league, or national championship, as you read about with UNC woman's lacrosse. That said, as a sport psychologist, my mission for athletes is always "the exceptional execution of extraordinary excellence." I call this "the X-Factor," the process which is achieved by diligent, eager attention to all "the little things," the essentials that can be controlled. This strong culture creates goals that are in the now, process oriented objectives that serve as beacons on the horizon that keep all of us on track, living the lifestyle of a champion. In this regard, practice sessions become tantamount to a championship game, whereby you set a high standard and demand from each other strict adherence to these standards each time you enter the arena of play.

- Know that this journey, this "way," is filled with obstacles. You will lose and you will fail. Yet this process is open to teach you how to go to the next level. The obstacles become challenges that you courageously embrace as opportunities to be tested, to learn, and ultimately to forge ahead. Plateaus will appear, and rather than get impatient or frustrated, you use these times to adapt to that level, master it, and go on to discover levels beyond what you thought were limits. To force or try to push yourself past the plateau will prove to be futile, counterproductive, and discouraging. Plateaus are simply one more natural stop on the journey, time to refuel your emotional, spiritual, mental tanks, enjoy the moment, accrue the confidence from mastering that level, and then advance not when you think you should, but when the time is right. Trust that when you go slower, you often arrive sooner.
- Athletes in such a culture refuse to offer excuses when they experience slumps, choking, and blocks, or have a mental meltdown, in their performance. They expect fluctuations and listen to their song. In a safe, sacred environment (team and inner self) they will continue on the road to peak performance and mental toughness. Remember that excuses are regressions, failures,

mistakes. They allow the mind to "check out," not care, and justify failure and write it off as useless when, indeed, it is our guru, teacher, mentor...how we learn all that we know. Embrace and accept failure— this builds mental toughness and team cohesion.

In alignment with all that has been said above, take a look at these Ten Building Blocks of strong, heart-directed cultures and imagine ways to incorporate them into your system, if you haven't already done so.

1. COMMITMENT (to a higher cause, purpose, other than any one individual athlete or coach)
2. RESPONSIBILITY (accept your role as a significant one with you as a valued contributor)
3. ACCOUNTABILITY (give and take criticism as a path of growth and improvement, not a personal slight)
4. INTEGRITY (narrowing the gap between what you say and do)
5. RESPECT (game, opponent, self, coach, team)
6. TRUST (self, others, coach...our intentions are pure)
7. LEADERSHIP (everyone's work)
8. COURAGE/COMPASSION (see section on *The Lens of Compasion*)
9. SERVICE (sacrifice/suffering and focus on giving, not getting)
10. HUMILITY (give others credit, gratitude, and thankfulness for having been blessed with this opportunity).

Individually, athletes on such teams must be accountable by demonstrating their virtues/values/traits, and sport itself presents constant opportunities to cultivate this inner, spiritual development for athletics, and more so, all of life. Some of the other virtues/values/traits are: fearlessness, audaciousness, relentlessness, tenaciousness, patience, perseverance, persistence, flexibility, fortitude, and belief in self and others. My experience tells me that such virtues are often more vital than talent when trying to experience success.

Let me end this crucial segment by offering a definition of culture that helps to guide me in my team building process with athletes at the collegiate and professional levels. This may help you to focus on the big picture, a vision of what can be.

- Culture is who we are and how we do things "around here."
- Culture is about socially transmitted behavior patterns, beliefs, thoughts; these are the traits of the "Culture of Champs."
- A set of predominant attitudes/behaviors that characterize the team.
- Developed through education/mentoring/example.
- An atmosphere and environment that is welcoming, nurturing, that we create using the 10 Blocks and certain virtues.
- Culture works together to arrive at a common understanding that benefits all rather than one.
- It's a bond—not essential to be "best friends": (although this is often the outcome) yet crucial to accept and respect others' interests, strengths, and weaknesses.
- Shared experiences—resembles a family.
- Leadership in a culture that is healthy when it becomes

everyone's job. Leading is when you reflect the culture you create.

- Ritual—all healthy cultures create ritual, be it pre-game, practice, meditation/visualization, post-game. What is yours?

This segment was quite long. However, it is a most essential component of the coaching with heart journey. If you'd like to expand upon this you may want to peruse Part Four of my book, *The Way of The Champion* on team unity.

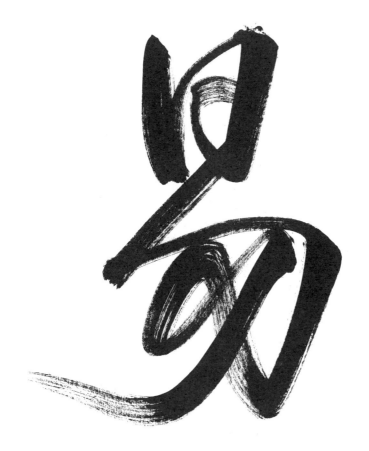

CYCLES OF CHANGE

The *Tao Te Ching* encourages us to notice the changing cycles of life. Welcome and respect these changes as they are inevitable. In Chinese, the words *I Pien* suggest that we stay in tune with the universal rhythm of nature that renews itself in cyclical fashion. We simply need to notice the cycles and act in harmony with them.

Change in sports is such a constant; change in teams where athletes graduate or get traded, change in national champions, change in coaches. Know that seasons change, moods shift, some days you're on, others you're off, you win then you lose, you're hot, then not. Nothing in sport or life is static. Peaks, ebbs, mountains, and valleys are nature's way. Accept and adjust to what you have been given.

We are reminded of this vast shift in life by the mythological phoenix that descends into its own ashes yet quickly rises up, expressing the exuberance of a new life. The wise heart-directed coach embraces with enthusiasm, the cycles of change, learning from the ups as well as the downs, never using change as a reason to distrust the system that's in place. Such a coach sees all change as a teacher and challenging opportunity to develop a strong sense of inner self.

Athletics, like life, is a constantly moving pendulum, a never-ending process constantly recycling itself as it gains eternal life. If you don't like a situation, know that, in time, it will change. All you can do at any moment is focus not upon what's changed but on what you have and how you will make the most of that, doing the best you can as a coach to get the most out of your players. Discover the gem inside the darkness.

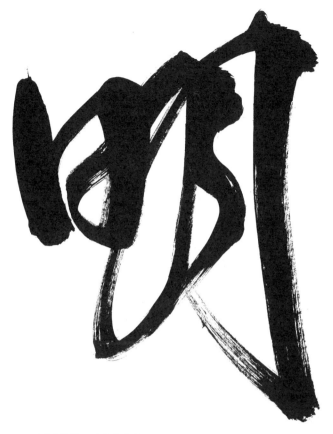

SHED LIGHT, SHOW PATH

Y ou may recall in *Like Frying a Delicate Fish* my reference
to the words of Confucius: a great leader "guides others and does not pull them along; urges them to go forward
by opening the way, yet refuses to take them to the place."

Along these same lines of thought, the *Tao Te Ching* suggests that good leaders "use little intervention as possible,
no manipulation or coercion. Shed light to show the path.
By so doing you guide by illuminating the way."

This is the way of leaders who coach with heart, using
guidance in place of control. As the Buddha knows, if you
truly want to control, let go of control—give more space for
athletes to grow, explore and find a way to discover their

own greatness. Know that control blocks self-reliance, vision, and creativity. For example, if you are an expert fisherman, rather than catch fish for the village and teach them to become dependent on your presence, try to guide and free them by teaching them how to fish, so they will always have food in your absence. With athletes, you want them to be creative and do it themselves while alone on the field or court. Guidance without excessive control is the way to help others realize their potential.

The Chinese symbol for control honors the way of letting be, allowing nature to prevail through loving guidance. Only when you are willing to let go of excessive control and micromanagement will you, your team, and others enjoy true learning and victory.

I have learned the following six strategies from my work with extraordinary coaches and these will help you to become a more conscious, heart-directed leader, guiding your athletes to places they never dreamed possible.

1. Be open to listening to criticism from others, particularly if it is the opinion of the majority. As a coach, corporate executive, or head of a household, show others your openness to feedback by asking them periodically (especially during times of tension and disharmony) to respond in writing to the question: "If you were in charge and had complete freedom to handle things your way, what would you do and how would you do it?" They should respond to this question anonymously, in order to ensure honest and truthful responses. They will respect and admire you for this, especially if you initiate positive change based on their suggestions

and criticisms.

2. Create an open, positive environment where all feel accepted, respected, and able to grow as individuals. With regard to the guidelines for team or group conduct, be consistent. Be sure to allow freedom for them to develop and be themselves.

3. I know I mentioned this previously, but before you criticize those you lead, first look for ways to give them credit. For example, you can say, "Sonia, I love the way you always hustle. Now, if you want to kick it up a notch, use your hands like this, and shuffle your feet at the same time." By the time you criticize her arm and footwork, she is ready to listen, knowing you acknowledge her work ethic. Be sure to provide concrete, specific data for your critique. Avoid gross generalizations such as "you always" or "you never." Search for ways that you, together with the athlete, coworker, or family member, can address the problem. Suggestions coming from them will hold more weight, and compliance will come more easily. When feasible, don't criticize during a performance. Your comments will be more effective if you wait and introduce them at the next practice session or on the next day.

4. As a coach or team leader, you need to understand that your position is only as strong and secure as you make your athletes feel. The players or workers can make or break you.

5. Avoid manipulation at all costs. As a leadership style, it creates anger, resentment, and loss of respect on the part of those it's used against. Power plays, trying to exert your position over others, and being "the boss"

are forms of manipulation that create environments of distrust and suspicion. Motivation and team spirit diminish with the use of such tactics.

6. The "Golden Rule" in Chinese is called "shu," meaning reciprocity and is written with two words "heart" and "alike." Simply stated it says do not do unto others what you would not have others do unto you (again, recall my reference in *Like Frying a Delicate Fish*—notice how all of this is inter-related). It is believed that if you follow this rule, your problems will be minimized. Harshness gets you nowhere. Why use it? When you are kind to others, you win their hearts and cooperation, which is what you really want and deserve. Taoist wisdom reminds us how the rulers of great societies governed without harshness. The coaches of great teams, I have noticed, guide with humane benevolence while leading within the understood parameters and boundaries of the culture. A child will always rebel against a harsh, unloving parent. This is no different than a coach and athlete. Life is a reciprocal adventure. If coaches work with athletes in the same way they wish their superiors to work with them, everyone is happy.

In these six ways you nourish your athletes. The *I Ching* clearly tells us that when the rulers nourish the ruled, they will watch them bring out their talents. With those who coach with heart, when their work is done, their leadership fulfilled, the athletes will feel, to paraphrase the *Tao Te Ching*, that they have done it themselves. Then we as coaches will realize how wonderfully effective we have been.

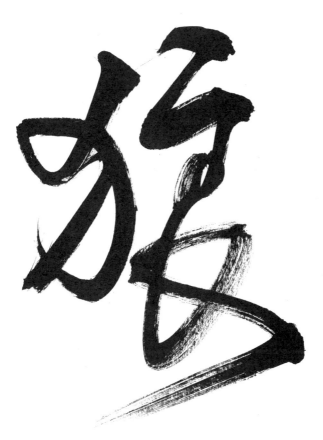

TWO WOLVES FIGHTING

What I have noticed in my coaching is that my single most limiting factor to my success is my internal negative self-judgment. If I feel I am good, I am good; if I feel no good, I act ineffectively. My thought process either strengthens me or weakens me. Thoughts have an energy of their own. For example, if my thoughts conflict with the direction I wish to go or what I wish to create with my team, the thoughts win.

Every one of us has both negative and positive thoughts in our minds, and at the same time. It's like having two different wolves inside fighting incessantly. The negative wolf claims that I am ineffective, not valued, afraid, uncaring; I call this "stinking thinking." The positive wolf, on the other hand, states that I am effective, caring, compassionate, courageous, and strong. I call this "confident thought." When the battle is completed, the wolf who is victorious is the one you feed. The idea is to recognize the confident thought patterns and to use them creatively to your advantage while disregarding those that make no sense.

As described in this book (see segment *Strength of Ten Tigers*), meditation is one effective way to help you focus on positive thinking; affirmations are another. Who you are, what you do, and where you go, are the direct results of the thoughts you choose. In sports, your effectiveness as a coach is shaped by your mind; you become what you think. For example, let's say one of your athletes gets unraveled after a poor performance. Her thoughts are: "I stink. What's wrong with me? I can't win." These words create self-doubt, and she begins to compete tentatively out of fear of losing. If instead she says to herself: "Yeah, that was an awful performance, but I can do better. I'm a strong, elite athlete. Here I go," her more positive, proactive affirmation would guide her to resume playing in a more focused way. When you change your thought, your performance follows. When you are coaching or recruiting, notice the difference in how you feel about your capabilities when you think, "I can do it—I am a good coach" versus "I can't do it—I'm the worst." Shifting between negative and positive thoughts creates a subsequent shift in your moods and subsequent behavior. When evaluating your performance, rather than focusing on negative stinking thinking—"What's wrong with me?"— ask yourself "What's right about me?" This second question is a proactive thought that creates forward movement and

confidence. We are all responsible for our own mental freedom. Ask yourself: Is my glass of thoughts half empty or
half full? I choose to think positively and ask, Why not? I
change my outlook and performance by focusing on possibilities, not disabilities.

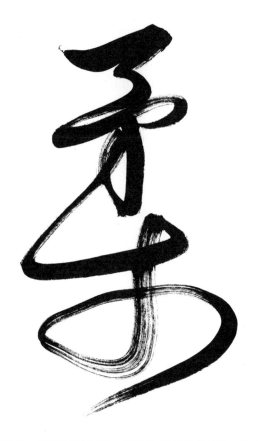

SOFTER EFFORT, STRONGER RESULT

The most yielding parts of the world
Overtake the most rigid parts.
That which is most tender
Can penetrate continually.

Lao-Tzu believed that little soft streams create massive strong rivers. Subtle efforts yield amazing outcomes. Soft is, indeed, strong in most aspects of good leadership. It is the equivalent of "tender strength."

Coaching athletes with heart is to expose them to the notion that on many occasions a softer effort produces greater results. We often talk about "letting the game come to you" rather than being hard and forcing, pushing and making it happen.

Softer approaches to leading others mean to "get out of the way" and refuse to micro-manage the path of your ath- letes. Communicating in a softer, yet direct way helps ath- letes to listen and follow because they feel respected and loved.

You may think that a soft muscle is a weak muscle, yet the opposite is true. Try executing five pull ups with your arms tight and hard. Take a minute's pause, make your muscles soft yet firm and repeat the process. Do you notice the difference? Softer, more relaxed muscles are more compliant and effective. In a sense, they are stronger, as you will be when more relaxed and a bit less edgy.

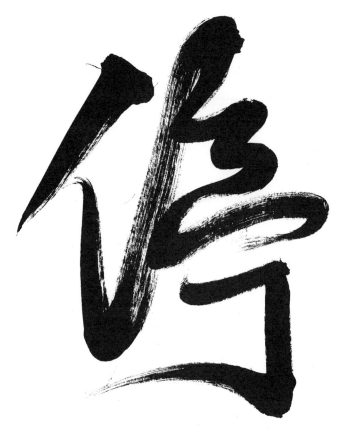

HASTE MAKES WASTE

The Tao reminds us to observe calmly the natural unfolding of events. Rapid growth and advancement, be it in athletics or life, is unnatural. Hold on to your inner hopes, dreams, and vision in the gradual flowing of you and your team's potential. Enjoy the moment of waiting to be, yet simply be here and now. Lao-Tzu encourages patience and mentions how all things occur at their appropriate time. Patience is the willingness to enjoy and immerse yourself in the process, the flow of life, as it assumes its own form and shape.

What we are talking about here is the entering of a new time zone, one where slowing down is faster than speeding up. You have often coached or heard of athletes who want to take the fast train to the top only to experience burn-out, illness, injury, and unforeseen obstacles along the path. Personally, I have experienced so may "over-use" injuries trying to get my body to respond too quickly to an unrealistic training program. Instead of getting to the next level in three months, what I had hoped for, I tried to accelerate the process and it took six months instead. I was a victim of the "hurry-up" sickness, too much, too soon.

When working with athletes, coach with your heart not your forcing, pushing mind. Your mind says to push, force, and make it happen. The heart knows that it takes time to develop the body and the capacity to endure the physical demands placed upon it. Listen to your athletes when they show signs of fatigue, illness, or injury and you will mitigate their tension and anxiety, emotions that exacerbate the problem. Avoid a "delay of game" penalty by heeding the *Tao* advice, slower is quicker.

Remember that in athletics as in all of life, things do not occur as we think they should but when the time is right. There is a natural flow to all events. Notice the flow and avoid the chaos when you try to hasten the natural way.

Think about the race between the tortoise and the hare. Through the inner spiritual qualities of consistent, deliberate, steady, slow movement, the tortoise arrives sooner than the faster, inconsistent, spastic, fatigued hare. Haste, more often than not, makes waste.

Be patient, stay calmly focused on the vision and enjoy the unfolding of things to come at the right time.

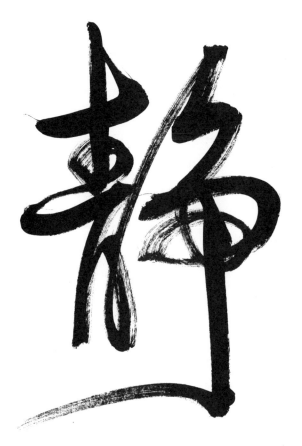

WEATHERING THE STORM

Just as the tumultuous chaos of a thunderstorm brings a nurturing rain that allows life to flourish, so too in human affairs times of advancement are preceded by times of disorder. Success comes to those who can weather the storm.

I Ching

Having worked with some of this nation's best coaches, I notice they have both an open-hearted acceptance for setbacks and admit openly to others that they fail and make mistakes. They learn from their mistakes, improve, and then succeed. My life has been a pattern of many losses, rejections, and failures, yet I know I am better because of such loss.

Failure is often associated with crisis. The word for "crisis" in Chinese means two things simultaneously: danger and opportunity. The really good coaches, although they do not like to lose, perceive and accept failures as opportunities to learn, and then go on as they forge ahead. My favorite question to ask the team after a painful loss is: why are we a better team today than we were yesterday before that loss? Once we examine this concept, we begin to embrace the importance of failure as success. Clearly, they are disappointed over the setbacks but they also realize it's all part of the journey, the bigger picture of human development and growth.

When athletes I coach experience failures, setbacks, and mistakes, I want to remind them that there are two types of performers: those who fail and those who will. Use these guidelines to help your athletes to accept failure as nature's way to help us learn and improve:

- Remember that it is absolutely impossible for any coach or athlete to be thoroughly successful, competent, and achieving. Failure is a part of the process of their ultimate success. Performance is a roller coaster, and to think otherwise is extremely irrational and the cause of much stress. Ups and downs can be expected. You win some, lose some; you're hot, you're not. Don't fight with yourself when failure, the teacher, pays an unexpected visit. Open up to learning from it.
- Mastery, as scholar George Leonard states in his important book by the same name, takes time. Patience, persistence, and perseverance are the three P's of per-

formance that will help propel your protégés to proper prior planning for extraordinary outcomes and results, as well as a deeper and more meaningful relationship with their sport.

- True failure can be defined as your unwillingness to get up when knocked down, and take the risks to grow and improve. Never look back with regret and wish you had taken the risk to go all-out only to find out how good you could have been.

- Change your expectations with regard to outcomes. They are setups for dissatisfaction. Like the Zen samurai warrior, expect nothing, but be ready for anything. Create solid preferences, and then do everything within your ability and power to bring those preferences to fruition.

- Failure is not the end of the world as we know it. No one ever died from it. But it does feel bad. When you look back upon outward success or failures in competitive situations, remember this: You are never as great as your best victory, and never as bad as your worst defeat. Refuse to give too much credence to your results.

I like to suggest to my athletes that they create affirmations to be used as touchstones to keep them on the right track. Create your own or tailor any of the following to your needs:

- The arrow that hits the bull's eye is the result of 100 misses
- Failures are lessons from which to learn

- Adversity leads to inner strength. I am a better athlete, worker, person because of it
- I act, not react; I learn from failure
- Setbacks are my teachers—they help me to go beyond my limits.

According to the *Tao Te Ching*, in the natural law, "we lose and in this way gain." Success does come to anyone who is willing to weather the storm.

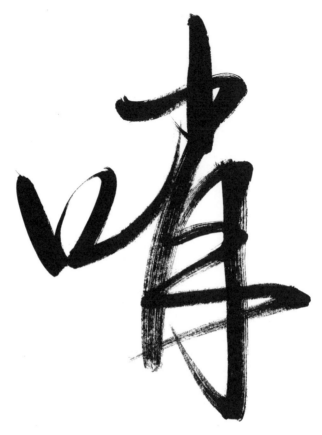

WHISTLES BLOWING IN THE WIND

Extraordinary leaders are those who
Reside in the background, merely visible, subtly
Influencing, commanding from a distance.

Tao Te Ching no. 17

So it is with those who coach with heart. They refuse to micro-manage and constantly interfere with the process and progress of their athletes. They use a subtle leadership, one that guides rather than rules. What I notice is how some coaches are overly visible and overbearing, especially during practice. I am certain that you are familiar with the kind of coach I call "Whistle Willy." Through a lack of trust in his or her athletes' ability to problem solve, to correct errors, and to be creative on their own, there is a sound of whistles blowing in the wind, stopping play and interfering with the natural flow of the practice session. I can understand when something is unproductive and repeating itself over and over that you may want to stop the action and use it as a teachable moment. But more than likely, it's best to let most situations play themselves out and when practice is over, call them together and point out constructive observations and make appropriate corrections. I have this belief that many coaches feel like they are not doing their job unless they are blowing the whistle. It becomes a distracting habit, at best, and worst of all, the athletes never get a chance to "figure it out" on their own. They become conditioned to having the coaches solve the problems. Before they know it, they forget what's been corrected because there were too many corrections being made.

The other disturbing aspect to the whistle is how it becomes a tool to "catch the athlete doing something wrong." When the whistle sounds, the athlete's body language, facial expressions, and grunts demonstrate a negative "vibe" that communicates: "Ugh, what's wrong now?" Or "this is ridiculous, let's keep playing." I wonder how the level of play would change if the whistle became the tool for "catching the athlete doing something right"?

I like to think about how being an excellent coach is like being a really good waiter. Imagine having an intimate dinner with someone who is important, someone special. In the middle of a tender moment, the waiter, unaware of this moment of intimacy, rushes by the table, stops, and in the middle of your sentence, interrupts to say: "everything all right?"

And you want to say "not really;" but let it slide. Or, how about when your mouth is full of food and the waiter asks how it tastes. Some waiters, like "Whistle Willy," are constantly visiting the table to correct a glass half-filled, or take a plate that still contains food. The constant interruption of the flow can ruin a perfectly good evening or a perfectly good practice session.

As a coach, I want to send a message to the athletes who I care for: I am there for them when things get out of control and I trust and respect their ability to take responsibility to make necessary corrections and resolve the problems at hand. I want to empower them to take ownership in their process of evolving as champions. If they really seem disjointed and chaotic, I can step in and lend a hand.

When I hear the State Farm commercial on the television, I think of this: Like a Good Waiter, Your Coach is There… only when you absolutely need assistance. Let them play, let them flow, let them have fun.

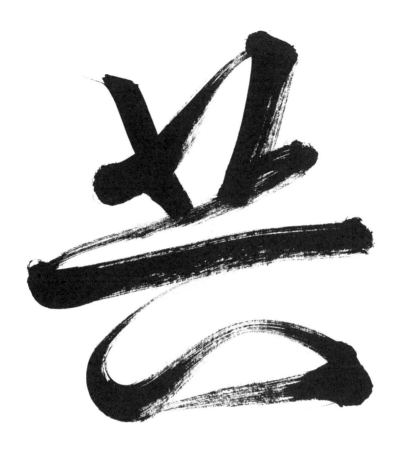

WORTHY OPPONENT,
SEEKING TOGETHER

Coaching with heart entails many things, one of which is having the ability to convince athletes to be worthy opponents who compete with heart, all out, giving their all and embracing the opponent who competes in like spirit in a relationship of giving and cooperation. It means forming an "unspoken partnership" of offering each other the best you have, to help bring out the best in each other. In Latin, the word for competition means "to seek together." In *Tao* terminology, it is called the *Worthy Opponent*.

I remember competing in a national 15K cross-country championship race in Houston, Texas. Many of the runners were talking about the ways they could defeat their closest rivals. They alluded to killer instinct and how important it was to beat the others. When I approached the pre-race favorite, I proceeded to shock him by saying, "I hope you have a great race." Confused by the words, the favorite inquired as to why I felt that way. I told him, "The better you run, the better I will, too." The favorite did win the race, and I claimed third, running my fastest time for the distance—and, in the process, pushing the winner to one of his greatest victories.

I was simply being a *Worthy Opponent*, helping the opposition to do well and running my best because of him. Because of this, our relationship grew stronger in many ways. Through his subsequent encouragement and kind words, I reached levels I never thought possible. We both got to know each other, our strengths and weaknesses, and used this information to race at higher levels together. I loved this opponent; why do so many of our athletes waste emotional and physical energy disliking those they compete against? Why focus on the opponent in this way? It may seem to help but in the long run an aware coach knows this approach is counterproductive, because anger, hate, and force diminish concentration, dilute energy, and lead to the downfall of the athlete.

Remember: change the mind and heart-set of your team. Have them view all athletic competitors as partners who, because of their outstanding work and performance, help them to understand themselves more fully and challenge them to step up and demonstrate their best. Begin to experience the powerful connection and relationship with any opponent in the world of competitive athletics and life. For example, see your workout buddies, your training partners, your colleagues, as a partnership. The better they perform, the better you will ultimately be. Feel the advantages in athletics of working together, with synergistic competition providing a surplus of energy for positive performance. Know your opposition in this new, refreshing way, not only as a competitor, but as a partner as well.

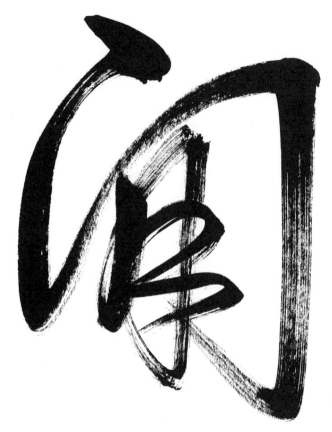

TAO OF LOA FING

Looking back upon all that I have written thus far, I realize I've been at it a while and I'm beginning to get a bit tired and worn down. I have been very busy with this project. Yet, I must mention to you, the importance of occasionally not being busy along the way. My experience working with coaches over several decades is that they find it difficult to separate themselves from their passion, as I have from my writing. The problem is, wonderful coaching is like eating your favorite food. If you have it every day, in time, you will come to dislike what you once loved. Let me elaborate further.

We have previously learned that *Tao* is the Chinese word

meaning "The Way," the way of nature, the way things were meant to be. I wish to suggest to all coaches the importance of showing yourself and your athletes the way (*Tao*) of Loa Fing, the not so Chinese word meaning to "chillax," to kick back, to simply loaf. This is nature's way. Great music is the result of the pause between the notes, rather than the notes themselves. The pause is what makes it what it is, otherwise you will just have noise. We need to consider the relevance of pausing in our athletic lives…doing nothing and having down time. In his classic work, *The Importance of Living*, Chinese scholar and author Lin Yutang, writes a whole chapter on "the Importance of Loafing." Now there's a word most of us in sports despise as well as those who practice it. Growing up, I learned early on that it is a serious offense to loaf—a major sin. Daydreaming was punished by the nuns in Catholic school. "Stop your daydreaming, Lynch" were common words uttered by these unimaginative souls. After all, I am here to tell you that everything I am today, every book that I have written, and my best work to date has all been the direct result of, yes, daydreaming while loafing. As an established and recognized professional in today's world, I must not let on that I love to loaf too much. After all, others will think I am not serious and therefore not "good enough" right? Wrong!

Too many people, coaches especially, whom I know want to look busy—this makes them feel important and that's okay. But this leads to complications. For me, I aim to be simply "busy enough," a healthy compromise between two extremes. In Chinese, the word for "busy" clearly means the killing or death of the heart. You draw your own conclusion. The only thing I want to be busy about is living. I want time to have lots of clients and meetings and appointments. My clients could be my family, my meetings may be with my friends as we run for hours in the wilderness, and my ap-

pointments can be with myself as I take the time to create, write, think, and design—a life that fits skin tight over my spirit. I also must shop for good nutritious food and cook lovely (filled with love) meals for those important others with whom I share my life. Then, I get to do my work and attend to my calling, with amazing open hearted people, athletes, and coaches, and give them the time they desire, choosing, of course, those who understand the importance of loafing. This is good leadership.

Daydreaming should be seriously scheduled in the class-room, boardroom, bathroom, and bedroom. As coaches, we may want to consider setting aside the time where we can meditate, and clear our minds. The better we all feel inside, the better our lives work outside but this takes time—time away from the maddening pace, the frenetic storm, and the closing down of our hearts so we can open them to a way of child-like discovery. That's what good leaders do, good ath-letes do, good parents do; what you will do, too, right?

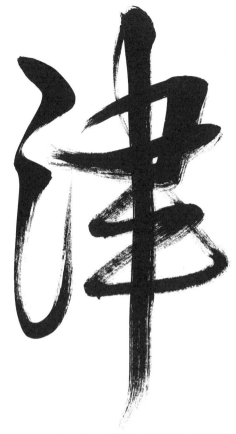

QUESTIONS ON THE QUEST

Here are a series of twenty penetrating questions that I use in my clinics and workshops to help coaches navigate deeper and wider into their quest to coach with heart. Don't rush to complete. Take some time to contemplate your responses and have fun doing so. There are no "right answers" or "best responses." Simply use these as guides that will give you more understanding about where you've been, where you are, and where you are going. Choose only those that seem most relevant. These work for your athletes as well. Simply substitute the word "athlete" for "coach."

1. What is the greatest misconception about you as a coach? How could you change it if you wanted to?

2. What has been your toughest moment on and off the court in your coaching career? What did you learn from it?

3. What has been your biggest disappointment as a coach so far? What can be done about it?

4. What are you most proud of as a coach?

5. If wishes could come true, what three would you ask for? What can be done to help bring these to fruition?

6. Looking back on your coaching career, is there anything you'd do differently? What could be done now?

7. When you are at your best as a coach, what contributes to it and how can you bring this to your trade more consistently?

8. What specific traits, characteristics, or qualities about you have helped you to get where you are?

9. Why can you be what you want to be?

10. What do you like best about your life as a coach?

11. What would help make your coaching more joyful, productive, and interesting?

12. What do you need to stop doing that you are doing now in order to be a better coach? What do you need to start doing that you're not doing in order to be a better coach? What do you need to continue doing that you are doing, in order to be the coach you are?

13. What regrets (specifically) could you have when your coaching days are over? What can you do now to ensure these regrets do not happen?

14. When all is said and done, what five specific words would you like others to use to describe you as a

person and coach? What specific things can you do (or how can you be) to increase the chances of this happening?

15. What one book has had the most influence on you and your life and how?

16. What message do you wish your athletes to send to your opponents? What do you and they need to do to make sure it gets sent and received?

17. Suffering and sacrifice are adverse conditions that bring opportunity for breakthroughs and advancement. What is sacrifice and suffering for you as a coach and how to you best cope with either?

18. What's going well with you and your team? What needs work and how will you handle it?

19. What excites you most about being part of your team?

20. What have been the three biggest accomplishments in your entire life and how does each impact you at this moment in time?

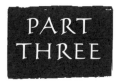

PART
THREE

WISDOM OF THE WATERCOURSE WAY

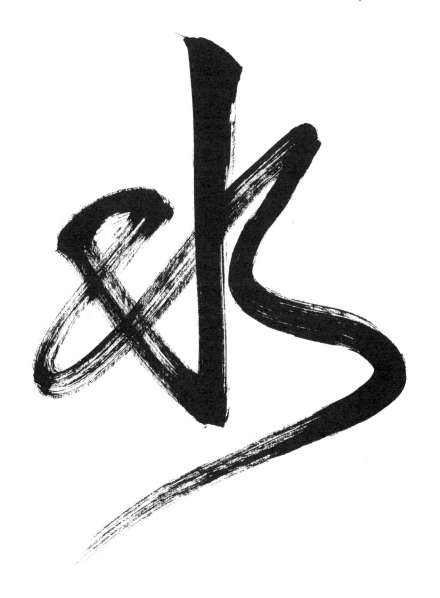

Tao is often referred to as the watercourse way. In fact, it refers to the fluid flow of nature and this flow of water is often used as a principal metaphor by Lao-Tzu and other Chinese scholars. For a Taoist, water is the basis of all life as it nurtures and nourishes all living things. It is the path of least resistance as you understand and flow with fatigue, loss, setbacks, and failures. It is soft yet strong as it can wear away stone and light up cities. Like the mind, water establishes clarity from stillness yet, unlike the mind, water requires no effort to do so. Human beings, it has been said, are at least 75% water and for this reason water becomes an important model for our behavior, especially with coaching. Coaching with heart is actually akin to pure, calm, and uncontaminated water. Uncontaminated hearts are made of pure, purposeful intention, free of wrong doing, and without harm, are clear, lucid and calm. Such hearts do not force but "go with the flow like H2O." The teachings and lessons outlined in this book from the *Tao Te Ching*, are water-like bits of wisdom pointing to the way of least resistance in all actions. It is referred to in Chinese as Wu Wei, the effortless effort. The Tao teaches that we can coach, mentor, and guide well by doing little and when all is done, those led will say "we have done it ourselves." Lao-Tzu, in verse #60 of the *Tao Te Ching* asks that the leader leads as one cooks a delicate fish, softly. The coach with a dancing heart leads without forcing and relies on understanding how to govern by observing the nature of water.

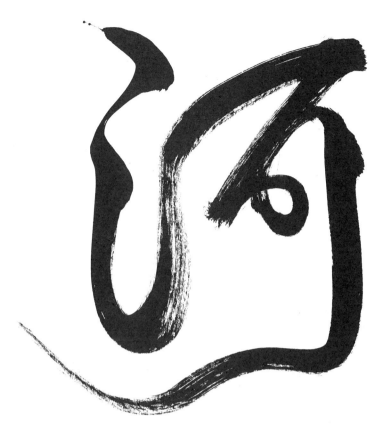

THE RIVER DANCE

The metaphor of flowing water is best exemplified by the unpredictable and continual dance of the river throughout its journey. The journey of this book is really not much different as once again, it is the image of such liquid that teaches us how to navigate the unchartered waters of our challenging professions. I simply ask that you trust the process just as you ask your athletes and any of those whom you lead to trust your process, believe in your system as you take and guide them along the path of personal and collective greatness and fulfillment.

This process is much like this dancing river which makes its way from high up in the mountains, down through the canyons, and empties into the vast waters of the open and receptive sea. The dancing heart journey of coaching, like the dancing river, moves slowly at times, faced with obstacles such as emotional or spiritual blockages. With clarity and understanding, the journey proceeds cautiously and finds openings where movement becomes accelerated, like the river rapidly increasing its speed through the narrows. At times, you will feel as though you are not making any progress along the way, like the river reversing itself turning in a different direction as if it has lost its compass. Yet like the river, you return on course carving out channels that enable you to fluidly flow in the desired direction. Your journey, like its watery counterpart, will have many reversals, setbacks, failures, and losses. All of this movement is a natural progression in your evolving process of being an extraordinary, heart-felt, athlete-centered coach. This is a process no different than what the athletes you coach experience. We are all in the same boat so to speak and this is the point where compassion for each other's journey takes place. Only the great coaches acknowledge, trust, and accept this natural process to be so. When you grow daisies, you would never think of pulling them up in order to accelerate their growth as they break through the soil for the first time. You trust that they will grow when ready, one millimeter at a time. Your coaching journey may also be slow. No need to panic or be fearful. After years of functioning in leadership and coaching capacities, I am still experiencing setbacks and failures, learning from them and continuing to go forward because I love the ride. It has been an amazing, continual journey of growth, fulfillment, and joy amid the setbacks and failures. There have been many roads, many choices, decisions and transitions. Somehow with my trust in the process, the universe (the *Tao*) has helped me along the path, placing well-positioned obstacles in my way to teach me yet another lesson. Because things don't always go as I wish they would, I stop and wonder if there is some greater lesson I need to learn. I keep going and wait for the best solution to reveal itself. I always seem to be okay when I trust and follow the signs presented to me along the way. I struggle when I don't.

To help you with the process, remember the following, and pass these on to your athletes as these will help them as well:

1. It's not about you, its' about them. This is an athlete-centered model.
2. Stay emotionally engaged to them; love them for their pure intentions.
3. Know the difference between what you can and cannot control. Hint: you can't control them.
4. Forget about outcomes and focus on the process.
5. Be real, be open, be authentic, be transparent, be receptive and be service oriented.

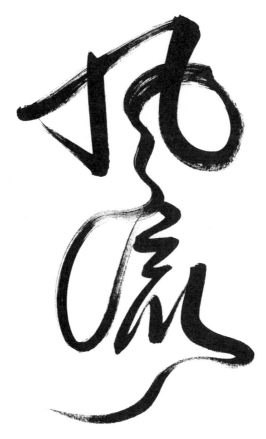

TRUSTFUL GUIDES ALONG THE WAY

I mentioned earlier in the book that I do not pretend to have answers, just some observations from my years working professionally in sports with extraordinary coaches and athletes. On this journey, you will learn the same way. You will observe and internalize that which works and that which doesn't. Like the river, you must learn to be a great coach through your ups and downs, your reversals, twists, and turns. And, along that river, there will appear certain practical gems to help you to trust and stay the course on the turbulent waters of extraordinary coaching. The following are several trustworthy "truths," or river guides, that will comfort you along the way. Write each one on a 3"x5" index card and flip through them during times of self doubt and discouragement; they will serve you well, acting as your "river guides" along the watercourse way.

1. Ancient Chinese wisdom states that the journey of a thousand miles begins with a single step. The task of changing your coaching can seem daunting. Begin by taking the first step and follow up with one step at a time. How do you eat an elephant? One bite at a time. Just try to implement a few of the book's suggestions and take on more as you become comfortable with those you've learned.

2. Once you begin a journey, never lose heart. Through steadfast perseverance, you will attain success. To help with this, focus on the joy of the journey, the process, rather than the goal. The experience itself is worthwhile.

3. Chinese wisdom, as I mentioned previously, tells us: "we lose and in this way, win." Understand that all of your mistakes, errors, setbacks, losses, and failures as a coach are your teachers. An old Zen Buddhist saying is: "the arrow that hits the bull's eye is the result of 100 misses." Learn from your loss and you will advance. All extraordinary things happen to ordinary people who choose to learn from setbacks.

4. Plateaus in your coaching life are a natural part of the process. Embrace them as natural, essential periods that provide deeper learning and mastery. So many coaches, athletes, parents, and business professionals become frustrated and fight times of plateau, feeling that they are not improving. This is counterproduc-

tive. Accept this stage as nature's way of helping you to master what you have recently learned. One day you will wake up and think that you've taken it to a higher level overnight when, indeed, it's been happening during the plateau phase.

5. Remember, rapid growth and advancement with anything in life is unnatural. All greatness takes time. Our coaching development occurs not when we think it should, but when it is supposed to—when the time is right. Be patient and stay focused on the flow of things. Sometimes it is wise to slow down in order to arrive sooner.

6. From little streams come big rivers. This old Japanese saying reminds us to attend to the little things when trying to accomplish our goals. When we do, the goals will be achieved. Remember to attend to your nutritional needs, attitude, positive mind set, and all the other things you can control. What are the "little things" on your journey of success in coaching and life?

7. Your beliefs are limits. Examine them and you will find ways to go beyond. Henry Ford once said: "Whether you believe you can or you believe you can't, you are probably right." By changing the inner beliefs of your mind, you can change the outer limits of your life. Do you ever hear yourself say, "I can't do that"? Change it to "I can" then search for ways that you can make it happen. Tell yourself: "I am strong, I can do it." Your language must awaken in you possibility, not limitation.

8. If you find yourself trying to be the best in anything

you do, forget about it. Don't be the best; be the best you can be. Being the best at anything is something you can't control. You can control, however, being your very best. This will relax you and help you to achieve your greatest dreams.

9. Are you committed to being a great coach? True commitment is essential if you want to achieve your goals. It is a matter of devotion to a cause; it is the ingredient that enables all of us to make strides on the journey. Until you commit, there is hesitancy. Once you commit, things begin to happen. By commitment, I mean the desire to do all that it takes to realize your dreams. The sky is the limit when you demonstrate consistent, never-ending commitment to what you desire to achieve.

10. When coaching your team during a competitive event, remember that competition in Latin means to "seek together." Review the suggestions in *Worthy Opponent, Seeking Together*. I recommend that you consider all of your competitors as partners who help each other to seek greatness. Notice how a good competitor is someone who will challenge you to discover your best. I love a workout buddy who will push the pace on a run or bike ride. I want someone to attack the hill with intent. This forces me to push beyond what I thought were limits. Some days, I am the one to attack with intent. Whether working out, or coaching a team by working together, you achieve so much more.

11. Remember the "musical pauses" with your team (see again *The Tao of Loa Fing*). Getting in physical or men-

tal shape, regardless of your sport or activity, is the result of the rest (pause) or space between the workouts and meetings. Your cellular structure is fragile and demands periods of rest. You must learn how to "nurture" your body and mind into shape as opposed to excessively forcing or pushing it there. Help your athletes to learn this. And apply it to your already overly busy life.

12. Buddhism teaches us the value of moderation in all things. Sports, exercise, fitness, business, and life usher in vibrancy and wellness that make for a healthier, happier life, yet, in excess, it can strip us of the vitality accrued. Moderation allows us to dance between any two extremes with great agility. Extreme approaches in sports, business, and life can lead to injury, illness, and burnout. Being really good at what you do is a delicate balance. Great coaches achieve this balance.

13. Do you know the difference between a good performance and a bad performance? Help your athletes to understand the difference. It's very simple: good performances always happen when you have no expectations, let it happen and trust things will work out. This causes you to relax and focus on the process, the things you can control. Bad performances happen when you try to control results, outcomes, have great expectations. Trying to control results is impossible and causes anxiety, stress, and tension. So let go of what you can't control (results) and focus on the little things that help you to perform well.

14. Remember this thought: the challenge is always with-

in, the opponent is always you and the reward is always deeply personal. You don't sing to get to the end of the song. Neither should you coach to just get it done. Focus on the joy of the process...minute by minute, day by day.

Trustful Guides
Along the Way

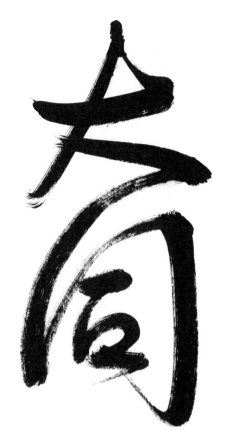

FLUID VISION FOR A GLOBAL MISSION

In this closing section, I wish to offer you a fluid vision of what can be when you take the risk to expand your every-day skill-set of coaching and choose an exciting and new array of tools and strategies. Change is not easy, yet the *Tao* reminds us that shift is inevitable. Risk is scary and creates an abundance of fear for all of us. Personally, I resist change, yet know deep inside, I need to take risks in order to continue to grow and expand in my profession and personal life. I think of author Ray Bradbury's idea of risk when he suggests that when standing at the edge of a cliff, jump, and build your wings on the way down—then you'll fly.

I also know that all significant change comes from within.

Begin to change and watch how your changes fluidly impact the lives of many others along the path. Notice that your creation is a fluid culture shift where athletes can be whole, authentic, and congruent with each other; the positive rela-

tionships that arise can change your world and give us a glimpse of what is possible in terms of outcomes, productivity, and satisfaction. Others see it, feel it, flow toward it, and want a part of what is happening. As that woman said in the restaurant observing Meg Ryan with Billy Chrystal in *When Harry Met Sally*, "I want some of what she's having." Coaching with heart is attractive; it's addictive; it feels so good. People relate to heart-driven energies; they crave it. We are all made up of hearts whether in athletics, business, schools, hospitals, churches, or families. We function and flow on a higher plane professionally and in life with Heart Chi, a way to be.

My vision is one that is a different, more dynamic and fluid way of being, one where there is an ongoing process consciously done within all structures or organizations where the mission becomes: "do all you can to be all you can be in order to realize your full human capacity." In order for this to happen, I offer a few suggestions for such a fluid global culture shift:

1. Leaders and followers must all be seen, viewed, and accepted as partners in a strong supportive environment
2. Consider the mantra: "Give Not Get" to establish an environment of pure selflessness and service
3. Praise and reinforce the power of intuitive guidance and decision making
4. Imagine how to integrate a group-wide meditation-

mindfulness practice on a daily basis. This is being accomplished nationwide inside athletic programs and corporations

5. Reinforce risk-taking and "outside-the-box" thinking as a way to create greater growth and expansion for yourself and those whom you lead
6. Try establishing a "Rule of One" philosophy: one person, one positive comment to them, one day at a time
7. Establish One Rule: "Do the Right Thing" and notice how this proactive (versus reactive rules: don't do this or that) statement encompasses all appropriate behaviors
8. Recruit "heart athletes" only: those who "buy-in" and wish to make a difference for themselves and others through service
9. Create a list of personalized (individual or group) "essential absolutes," behaviors or actions that others can aspire to, giving meaning, purpose, and identity to the group culture
10. Begin to create culture rituals as a way to define the shift in the organization, group, team, family. Celebration of birthdays, Friday evening dinners together, retreats, are but a few of the ways to manage this.

It will take courage to take the risk to make changes. It is the same courage that you demand from your athletes as they embark on their journey of competing with heart. Know that change is always a challenge yet refreshingly rewarding. You follow this vision by following your heart, believing that such a shift is what we all want, need, and crave. This is a very special and exciting time to be a coach. We are truly blessed with an important, vital calling where we can create safe environments where others feel free to open their hearts and then we can step inside and coach them to believing they can be something other than ordinary.

Imagine what coaching would be like if we led in alignment with the principles of *Tao*, the more natural way where a coach is humble, kind, non-judgmental, firm yet fair, intuitive, and selfless, encouraging positive focus and direction through modeling a more effective, enlightened style of leadership, where the spiritual virtues resolve conflict and contribute to harmony; where cooperation and partnership are honored for the purposes of human dignity; where coaches and leaders belong to the culture and not own it; where we can all blossom to our full human potential in an environment of unconditional positive regard. Let the wisdom and lessons in this book, guide and lead you to fulfilling such a vision.

Although this book is coming to an end, the journey for us to coach with heart is just beginning—like the symbolic circle, the journey never ends. I know I have mentioned this previously, yet I feel it is imperative to state it as it is written in the *Tao Te Ching*:

> *With good leaders*
> *When their work is done*
> *Their task fulfilled*
> *The people will all say:*
> *"We have done it ourselves."*